HOW TO BE A
babe

HOW TO BE A

babe

Overcome Your **Romantic Obsessions** and Other Obstacles to having the **Sex Life You Deserve!**

JOY DAVIDSON, Ph.D.

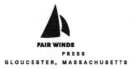

FAIR WINDS
PRESS
GLOUCESTER, MASSACHUSETTS

First published in the U.S.A. by
Fair Winds Press
33 Commercial Street
Gloucester, Massachusetts   01930-5089

ISBN 1-59233-005-3

Cover design and interior book design
by Laura McFadden Design, Inc.
laura.mcfadden@rcn.com

Cover image by Merton Gauster/Photonica

Printed and bound in USA

Acknowledgments

How to Be a Babe is not just my book, it is "our" book. Many people contributed to making it possible, making it real, and making it worthy of the reader.

Much gratitude to my agents extraordinaire, Marilyn Allen, Coleen O'Shea, and Robert Diforio. With enthusiasm, skill, and care, they midwifed the ideas contained in my original proposal and found them a home.

Thanks to the überBabes at Fair Winds Press. Holly Schmidt and Paula Munier "got it" from the outset, invited me in, and guided the project. With deep appreciation I acknowledge my editor, Wendy Simard, whose talent, clarity of purpose, and saintly patience saved me from myself on more than one occasion and contributed enormously to the final product.

Thanks to Janelle Randazza for her ongoing support, Barb Karg for copyediting with lightning speed and a light touch, Claire MacMaster and Silke Braun for art direction, and Dalyn Miller for media magic.

On the home front: I am one of the luckiest people alive to be surrounded by so much affection and talent. For reading and critiquing in the early stages as well as ongoing support, thank you to Annie Beckman, Jordan Buck, Debra Davidson, and Judie Fein.

For being there with valuable contributions and true caring, hugs to Becky Bay, Vena Blanchard, Patti Britton, Jack Davidson, Alex Delano,

Beverly Engel, Allena Gabosch, Jessica Hansberry, Shari Hanson, and Regina Leeds.

Gratitude to Stephen Gabosch for unwavering encouragement, storms of bliss, and soulful life lessons.

Special appreciation to Jordan Buck for being my lifeline and cheerleader in countless ways, day in and day out.

On the well-being front: Heartfelt thanks go to Kim Chodakauskas for aid beyond the call of duty, and to Stephanie Isch, Martha Panitch, and Eileen Stretch.

This book neither claims to create an entirely new theoretical framework for understanding intimate relationships nor to be a faithful representation of any existing system. I am indebted to others who have imparted their wisdom and clinical skill to me, either through the written or the spoken word. I have distilled what has been most useful into my practice, my life, and my writing. I wish to acknowledge family systems pioneer Murray Bowen and those who have explicated or expanded upon his theories, especially Michael Kerr, Harriet Lerner, and David Schnarch. I extend appreciation to the formal sexology community, whose research and cumulative efforts have given sustenance and backbone to my work. Just as importantly, I honor the pro-sex feminist activists who, over the past 20 years, have altered the sexual landscape through their take-no-prisoners brand of enlightened sexual revolution. They are my heroines.

Finally, many thanks to my remarkable clients, whose dedication and bravery hearten me in unpredictable ways every day.

Joy Davidson, Ph.D.
Seattle, Washington
February, 2003

contents

"Life is either a daring adventure, or nothing."
—*Helen Keller*

Foreplay

I'm forever dazzled by the way life is filled with synchronicities. The very day I sat down at the computer to begin the book that you're now holding in your hands, I received a poignant e-mail from a girlfriend who lives in another state. It seemed that her thrilling long-distance relationship with the man she'd met online five months before was careening toward a crash, and she wrote to me in a rare fit of tearful consternation. Maybe it was her unaccustomed degree of confusion, maybe it was the coincidental timing of her letter, and maybe I just empathized, but in any event, her last few sentences resonated with me:

"Should I save myself more grief and cut him loose? Do I want to keep trying to forge a relationship with someone who is irresponsible and makes me feel crazy when we're apart just for the sake of having someone who makes me feel so magically alive when we're together? I know you can't tell me what to do, but I sure as hell wish someone would!"

In her words I heard the echo of thousands of other women's voices—the letters from readers of my magazine advice columns over the past ten years, my own therapy clients, my other dear friends—who have found themselves sucked down into emotional quicksand in the course of relationships they'd hoped would bring them joy, and instead led to self-reproach and despair. By and large these were smart, savvy women, and while the details of their relationships differed dramatically, they displayed in common a yearning for passionate, electric love, and a corresponding striving to be true to themselves. Somehow, these two basic urges failed to complement one another; instead, they seemed to operate at cross-purposes. In their relationships—even their brief ones or one-night stands—women like my friend with the long-distance lover often felt they had to make a choice. The choice was him or me, and all too often, "me" was voted down.

As someone who has asked the same questions and worn the same pinching shoes as the women I describe (plus spent half a lifetime helping ease their pain), I can tell you with certainty that few of us find ourselves in romantic predicaments because we're desperate, dysfunctional, or self-destructive. No, the vast majority of us are hot-blooded, hopeful, full of life, and courageous enough to risk following our hearts and other pulsating body parts. Most of us still believe in happy endings, we believe in commitment, we just don't have a clear game plan for achieving the ends we seek or for keeping our power switch on when emotional exhaustion creeps over us. Ultimately, it's so much easier to unplug or give in.

Many of us wonder whether it's our basic attitude toward life that's all wrong. Maybe we should expect less, feel less, risk less? Yet even as we pose the question, we have to admit that we like the fierce qualities in ourselves that attract us to the more, shall we say, intense relationship situations. We like embracing our longings and our hungers and we'd much rather sharpen our edges than lose them. So where does that leave us?

We are left having to face the real problem—one that we can't altogether blame on ourselves. While "taking responsibility" is a primary tenet of the therapeutic and human potential movements—and many women will take that axiom so far that they'll accept blame for rain at a picnic—there is such a thing as taking too *much* responsibility. We need to stop and understand why we struggle in that netherland between wanting and having, between self-determination and self-doubt. And, while I could offer a complicated answer (and many others have), I can also pare down the message to its key elements: *Women don't get lessons in living loud and juicy as we grow up—we get lessons in fitting in.* We don't learn to self-determine, we learn to merge with others. We aren't encouraged to reach out to loved ones from a place of pure power—we're taught to fuse with those we love out of perceived necessity, and fear. As a result, those of us with an unquenchable thirst for experience often make pretty blatant mistakes in our sex and love choices.

For example, my friend Ellie hangs out with a sexually open, artsy crowd, so, to avoid being seen as a repressed geek, she sexes it up with new men before even an itch of desire erupts. No wonder her whispered appraisal of sex is, "Mostly, I can take it or leave it." If she doesn't wait to do it until her desire is piqued, how hot can it be? Even though her life looks iconoclastic, she does what's expected—without great enthusiasm.

Marla would love to live in Ellie's free-spirited world, but having been raised a New England blue blood, she too does the expected, putting off intimacy until she's certain he will respect her in the morning. Of course, every now and then she picks up a perfect stranger, boffs him for the thrill of it, and then kicks him to the curb—but that's her little secret.

And then there's Bette, who doesn't know how to leave relationships even after they become toxic. She's convinced that if she can come up with the right strategy, her difficult, self-centered lover—the bad boy who excited her wildly at first blush—can be sculpted into the sensitive partner she needs long-term. It never happens, but she keeps trying.

A more sedate contingent of women than Ellie, Marla, or Bette—those whose yearnings for adventure have been stifled and submerged, who qualify as so-called good girls and look like they absorbed the rules of the relationship game from the start—make just as many unintended blunders as their more daredevil sisters. The most drastic of these is hiding their authentic selves, lest they invoke the disapproval or rejection of people who have come to matter more than their own truths. They often hitch up early, have kids well before they're thirty, and put their families first, first, first. On the surface they look like they're living a dream life, but in reality, every day is a bargain made with the devil of self-sacrifice. I've written extensively for women's magazines devoted to this particular cadre of women, and I find it heartbreaking to see how often their real selves cower in shadows so thick that just to begin searching for them requires a truckload of floodlights and a busload of bravery.

I wrote this book because I understand all the struggles. I've been there with some and been witness to others, and I've made a career of trying to figure out what it takes to be the kind of woman for whom coming alive comes, well...naturally.

In *How to Be a Babe*, you'll find your guide to living large; kicking obstacles out of the way; and loving yourself enough to love others with passion, integrity, and good sense. My message stems from my unflinching belief that desire is more than what we feel on the way to the bedroom, it's the spark that ignites our very lives. Yet, in no corner of our world does that spark set fire to more confusion, acting out, or shutting down than in the erotic domain. Each time we yield to, or shy away from, our authentic erotic voice, we come closer to understanding the mysteries tucked away within ourselves.

I believe that embracing our sexuality and erotic spirit is an art form—one which is at the root of our ability to thrive as creative, empowered women. I also believe that learning to express our sexual selves without stalling in self-defeating relationships is a practical, learnable skill. This book is your guide to excelling in both the art and the skill.

The Birthing of a Babe

In my own life I started out with a big dream and lots of confusion. I grew up in what these days is known as a dysfunctional family. My mother was depressed and rarely left the house. The older I became, the more frightened I was of turning out like her. I had only one real-life role model, my mother's sister, who, unlike all the other women in our extended family, remained unmarried, had lovers, and actually left the town in which she was raised to move to New York City. She was brave and glamorous, but she wasn't around a lot, and so I found other role models in the books I read voraciously—on the average of one per day. I remember how I fantasized at age nine or ten of growing up to be the kind of woman who leaped off the pages of those books. I consumed them deep into the night, huddled under my blanket with a flashlight, listening for footsteps that would signal my mom or dad coming too close to my room. I didn't want to get caught and have my secret readings discovered—I needed the time, late at night, when my heroines could come to life for me in pools of golden light studded with dark printer's ink.

I read mostly grown-up books that I checked out of the library or pinched from shelves in my grandmother's den, choosing them carefully for the presence of imaginary women who thought the unthinkable and inspired me to want to grow up and run off on my own as quickly as I could. It's funny to think that their "unthinkable" is behavior we take for granted today. But it wasn't the actual standards of behavior that mattered, it was the fact that my heroines stood for standards of social misbehavior, breaking the rules and challenging the status quo, all the while remaining unflappably self-possessed and serenely beautiful. In their daring coolness, they were everything the real-life women I knew were not.

Of course, it was easy to be a fictitious social warrior. Being a genuine challenger, filled with contradictions on the inside, living in a world filled with paradox on the outside, and battling to make sense of it all, turned out to be another, more convoluted story. I've been working on understanding that story for a very long time. As I achieve a better grasp, I teach others what I know—and I love writing it all down for my readers to soak up.

One of the other things I love is turning convention on its head. I love when an idea that is taken for granted as belonging to the male cultural-machine is suddenly co-opted by wild-eyed female insurrectionists.

Words carry power. In the world of myth and magic, just knowing the name of your adversaries means that you have power over them. (Remember Rumpelstiltskin, the fairy tale in which the princess was challenged to guess the vicious little gnome's name, and if she could utter it, she would save her baby from his clutches?) Back in the seventies, the single mutinous act of creating a bridge between the girlish *Miss* and the male-identified *Mrs.* by divining a new designation, *Ms.*, was a demonstration of defiance that, with the stroke of a pen and using only two simple letters of the alphabet, brought the nations newly erupting feminist consciousness from the side streets to Main Street. Today, it's strange to think that there was a time when *Ms.* didn't exist at all.

As word transgressions go, one of my favorite feminist usurpations is developed in the book *Cunt*, by Inga Muscio. I'll share a few jewels from Muscio's writing later, but for now, suffice to say that the point of the title is to transform a reviled, face-scrunching, "nice-girls-don't-say-that" word into a woman-loving, self-loving manifesto.

In *How to Be a Babe*, I've plucked a term from the vocabulary of female objectification—after all, being a babe is really about being cute and sexy and essentially brainless—and reclaimed it for smart and feisty gals everywhere. By no means does the reinventing of *Babe* compare with the inventing of *Ms.* or confer the shockingly subversive quality of *Cunt.* Still, I have to admit getting a kick out of kidnapping this mildly objectifying, conformist term, turning it on its head, and repackaging it laced with female dynamite.

What follows is the story of how this particular word evolution came into being.

A BABE AND PROUD OF IT!

Some years ago, I was in a relationship with a much younger man. After I met his best friends for the first time, he breezily reported that they had unanimously voted me a babe. "That's it?" I said, irritated. "That's *all* they said?" Frankly, I don't know why I expected more—these were *guys*, after all! My honey looked at me, amused. He shook his head sadly. "You don't get it do you? That's the highest compliment they could have paid you." He was so sweet in soothing my slightly ruffled and embarrassingly mature feathers that I quickly decided that when you're eighteen years older than your boyfriend, and his buddies still think you're a babe, you're better off shutting up and heaving a sigh of relief. It could have been far worse—they could have made crude remarks about the fact that this chick was old enough to have hatched him herself. *Babe*...yeah, I'll put that in the bank, thank you very much. By the time I went to bed that night, a sly smile graced my face. I wouldn't have admitted it, but I liked being a babe!

The truth is that nearly every woman, in some secret corner of her psyche, wants to think of herself as a babe—an attention-getter, an object of desire. Being a babe means we exude at least one kind of power that draws others to us. Maybe it's superficial, maybe it's male defined, maybe it's crude and politically incorrect, but running scared from truth never gained us an inch, and facing it always does.

Here's another truth as I see it: As women, we're raised to want to be wanted. We yearn to be desired with an urgency that fills us to near overflowing. Yet, being wanted can never be enough to satisfy us. If that's all we know of desire, we are at the mercy of those who do the *wanting*. Being wanted is a passive state—only one-half of a linked pair of cravings that generate real passion. The feeling that completes us is derived from the other partner in the intricate dance of desire—the wanting and the getting. We want to inspire desire, and we want to feel desire, feel it down to our bones, feel it with no apologies, feel it like thunder and watch it spill over into raging tempests of satisfaction.

When I decided to write about this aspect of femaleness and more, imagine my surprise when my publisher suggested a title that contained the word *babe*. How synchronistic! The more I chewed on it, the more enamored I was with the term's ability to embody *female* quintessence in female terms—to whisk it beyond its link to certain midriff baring, soft drink pedaling pop stars and their everyday imitators, and speak of passion and power in one breath.

Babe, Defined

Babe seems to embody a contemporary archetype, a woman made up of facets so complex, varied, and sometimes contradictory that they couldn't have existed all of a piece in our collective consciousness until this very moment in time. As the concentrated essence of babeness sprang to life in my mind, I could see her—the pure undiluted Babe—part revolutionary, part traditionalist, part sexual adventurer, part self-ordained goddess. Being a Babe conferred an aura of audacity and animalism; of authenticity and boldness; of balance, of bemusement, of self-determined eroticism. A Babe is who we get to be when we unclip ourselves from the leash of convention and let the most fearless, committed, and excited parts of ourselves storm forth. I realized that the little girl who fell in love with bookland heroines all those years ago was really slipping into Babeland. All my wannabes were Babes.

I pitched the idea to a few friends, but some had trouble with the notion of co-opting standard English. Then there were the surprises—the women who really got it—satire and seriousness all rolled into one.

"I wish someone had taught me how to be a Babe when I was in my twenties," said my forty-something physician pal. ("It's never too late," I countered. You won't catch me setting an age limit on Babes!) But my favorite response came from a friend who is a far too dedicated, hard-core radical feminist to find any redeeming charm in being a man-magnet, hair-tossing babe. She said:

I don't want to be anyone's Babe, but I wouldn't mind being my own. There's that moment in the morning, when I look in the mirror, and I think, she's pretty fucking cute. It's simple, it's objectifying, and it's totally liberating. For that moment, I'm a Babe, not only in the sense of self-regard, but as someone who feels she can be loved, admired, adored—someone who has this glow that's not just about looks at all, but that lifts up the people around her. There's an assertive confidence in thinking 'Hey, I'm a Babe!' Knowing I'm a Babe, I can kick out the boy or girl I just slept with who is jerking me around after sex, playing on my fears. I'm a Babe, and I don't have to take this shit! Its powerful, mostly because, on some level, its something we all want very badly: to own our wanting and let it rise and fall by itself. This is a kind of grace."

Yes, there is a certain grace in being fully responsive to ourselves. And although it doesn't start out being easy—and, by the way, it never gets really easy—being a Babe means staying committed to one's self. A Babe doesn't take shit. She develops boundaries—lines drawn in the sand— places she won't go, conventions she won't buy into, conformist rules she won't adhere to, principles she won't betray. A Babe admires who she is, and who she keeps becoming. A Babe unfurls herself like a sail, ever so slowly, all her life, and glides gracefully into the wind.

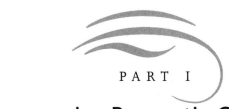

PART I

Overcoming Romantic Obsessions

CHAPTER 1

The Fine Art of Becoming a Babe

Be smart, be yourself, speak up, sex often

NOT LONG AGO, I was out to dinner with a small group of girlfriends and, as women naturally do, we began talking about our most recent struggles and conquests in relationships, our day-to-day lives, and the perpetual project of contending with ourselves—our own "stuff." In the course of this unguarded conversation, we each revealed strengths and frailties and secret wishes about who we'd like to be if only we could wave a magic wand and improve ourselves in an instant. "You know," said one of us, "if we all hopped into a blender and got someone to flip the switch, when they poured us out they'd find one hell of a perfect woman!" The rest of us screamed with laughter. Yes, together we had it covered! Although none of us is perfect, each contains enough pieces of perfect to produce a mind-blowing blend.

Becoming a Babe doesn't guarantee we'll become perfect either, although as you develop your Babeness you'll certainly feel more *perfected*. Even the women I consider the epitome of Babeness aren't perfect. In fact, part of the art of becoming a Babe is to accept your imperfections. My friend Darlene has this down.

At a glance, you wouldn't say of Darlene, "Wow! Now there goes a Babe!" She doesn't dress in a particularly fashion-forward or sexy way, though she does have her knock-out dress-up days. Her hair is still the same wavy chestnut that fringed her face at birth, and by supermodel standards she's seriously overweight, though anyone with a less jaundiced view can see that she looks simply delicious. Darlene is no vixen, yet she always seems to have a great guy in tow. In fact, she has had a very special partner for the past three years, and when you see the two of them together, their mutual devotion seems to rise off them like steam. There's plenty of heat in their intimate universe, too. Darlene takes to sexual experimentation like the proverbial duck to water. She loves her own body even with its imperfections and loves being pleased by her man. In the bedroom, there are no stringent rules except those that she and her honey divine from each moment of erotic inspiration.

Darlene's life isn't perfect, either—not by a long shot. She struggles with fibromyalgia, which makes exercise literally a pain. Last year, she lost her job during the last gasp of the sweeping dot-com bloodbath. Although she's working as a Web designer now, she was unemployed for quite a while and she hasn't yet settled into the groove of her career. Money has been tight, but Darlene often remarks that times have been far tougher for other people, and she never feels sorry for herself.

BABE BOOSTER

Be your own dominatrix. Keep a supply of gags in pretty colors on hand for those times when your nasty inner critic won't shut up.

Darlene possesses the enviable gift of being able to take bumps in the road in stride because she approaches change with a sense of openness and possibility. She believes that something exciting always extrudes from what was. Darlene is no Pollyanna, but she is still wide-eyed about life, and in some ways, she's more like sixteen than her actual thirty-one years, while in other ways she displays the maturity of a woman twice her age.

Darlene has a solid grasp on the idea that being who she is carries a lot more weight when it comes to her long-term happiness than does trying to fit in for the sake of making others comfortable. She has no interest in being anyone but straight-shooting, straightforward Darlene. She's flexible, she's compassionate, but she's no pushover and she's always one hundred percent real. And that's a big part of what makes Darlene a superstar Babe. Pick her up in a helicopter and drop her down anywhere you like—the middle of an antiwar rally, a dinner at the White House, a church supper, or an orgy—and the authentic Darlene will do just fine. Even if her boyfriend, whom she loves deeply, were to up and leave her without warning, she'd grieve and then she'd move on, armed with all the meaningful lessons she could extract from her heartache.

Darlene is a Babe because she hums a melody she composes herself— a brand new song each day. She'll never win a Grammy for her sounds, or get to shake it up in a thong on stage with a chorus of hip-swiveling, tap-dancing cuties, but she'll still be a Babe when she's eighty. There's no outside limit to the Babe power she'll amass in her lifetime, or the people she'll hearten by just being present. To my mind, that's success of extreme magnitude, and it's better than being perfect.

The ABCs of Being a Babe

Darlene wasn't born a Babe. Her childhood was stained by her father's departure for parts unknown when she was four, and by her mother's subsequent battle with the bottle. Today, one of her brothers is doing time for peddling drugs, the other is a career military man. Darlene's history could have given her plenty of classic justification for beginning a downward spiral or taking solace in rigid conservatism, but Darlene saw the impact that self-defeating choices have on one's life—she vowed not to let disappointments or even betrayal force her into self-destruction as her mother had, and she swore to be smarter and more loving than her incarcerated brother. She believed she could carve out a life of meaning and hopefulness despite the obstacles, and when all is said and done, that's what really makes her a Babe.

If Darlene could become a Babe, any woman can. Yes, it's a project. Becoming a Babe is real work, and we're not talking about eyeliner and spandex here! Becoming a Babe is hardly as easy as A-B-C, but it's as accessible as B-A-B-E. The word itself is the key to making a Babe's most empowering qualities attainable to each and every one of you.

BABE stands for:
 B Balance
 A Authenticity
 B Boldness
 E Eroticism

Let's examine these concepts one by one.

B IS FOR BALANCE

A Babe is a loving creature. She seeks to give, take, and express love. But love is a complicated concept, made even more so by the competing drives within us that vie for control over how we experience and express love.

On the one hand, we feel a drive to connect, to be close to others. On the other hand, we yearn to be individuals, self-contained and self-possessed. When we strike a healthy balance between these two drives, they complement one another beautifully, like two distinct but harmonious voices that give greater strength to a musical passage than either could achieve alone. But when just one of these drives dominates, love may be held hostage to its overwhelming force. For women, the *togetherness drive* usually rules, and when we love, we risk losing pieces of ourselves to our relationships.

The pattern builds slowly. We usually let go of one sliver of self at a time, until all the tiny slices add up to a huge chunk of our identities. Imagine yourself inside this sequence: First you let your lover choose the movie; then you say, sure, Thai food sounds great, even though you really want Italian; eventually, you feel undesirable when your guy is even slightly inattentive; and then, when you make love, you don't dare question his perfunctory three minutes of tongue titillation—in fact, you wonder if he's done you a big favor by venturing down there at all!

> **BABE BOOSTER**
>
> *Approach a relationship from the mind of a tightrope walker! There's a fine line between me, him, and we, and if you can walk the line, you won't plummet to the ground.*

The drive to be an individual impels us toward achieving difference from others, toward sustaining our own beliefs, values, and avenues of thinking. The sense of being a self-possessed, worthy individual is behind the ability to say something as basic as, "Honey, your mouth on my clit feels wonderful—please don't stop until I come!" Yes, these big concepts affect the tiniest efforts we make—or are ashamed to make—toward giving and getting satisfaction.

Holding onto yourself by attaining balance between loving attachment and respectful separation is the key to Babe power, but it's a quality that's far more easily identified than achieved. Among therapists, an individual's ability to be simultaneously close to her partner and self-possessed is known as *differentiation*. When we are differentiated, we remain sure about our own boundaries and priorities and we continue to act on them, though we are respectful of our partner's wishes, too. We simply don't allow his emotions—especially *his* anxieties—to bleed into us so that they overrun or become ours, and we don't allow our fear of loss or disapproval to bar us from speaking our truths.

Unfortunately, few—males *or* females—differentiate very well. Men are more likely to lean too far toward detachment, not because they need love any less than women, but because they're more terrified of dependency. Extreme disengagement is the flip side of extreme attachment, and neither are balanced places. We women fall all over ourselves wanting to merge, so much so that sometimes we can't tell where our psychic space ends and our lover's begins. Jokes that make sport of clingy women who say things like, "I'm cold—go put on a sweater!" are funny because they ring of an awkward truth.

Obsessive romances—the dramatic, seductive, gooey, juicy relationships we'll be talking about in the next chapter—obscure your ability to love honestly or even have the kind of light-socket sex you deserve. Obsessive romances represent the height of undifferentiated merging, a state we call *fusion*, where dependency is disguised as true love. Fused romances are disempowering romances, no matter how thrilling or compelling they may seem. Obsessive relationships thrive on our temptation to suck others' feelings inside ourselves, to make them more important than our identities or self-respect.

You can't maintain balance and be in an obsessive relationship—they're mutually exclusive qualities. Balance is also the cornerstone of our individual and erotic freedoms. The more sexually exploratory, daring, and demanding you'd like to be (or think you *might* like to be), the more balance you'll need to dredge up from within. As we move through the next two chapters, you'll see how balance can be achieved no matter how fused your relationships have been in the past. A Babe can get beyond fusion. In fact, a Babe can pretty much get beyond *anything*!

Understand, though, that balance isn't something you develop in a couple of weeks or by doing a few exercises in this or any other book. I won't kid you: It's a serious, ongoing process. It's going to be up to you to keep your dedication afloat long after you've turned this book's final page. But you'll discover very quickly that every ounce of work is worth the sweat, because once you begin this process, your world will literally turn inside out—you'll share yourself, but you won't give yourself away. You'll even share the best of yourself, but you'll accept no less from your partner in return.

A IS FOR AUTHENTICITY

A Babe is authentic. She doesn't bullshit herself, and she doesn't bullshit people she cares for. A Babe doesn't make a practice of telling little white lies—whether by commission or omission—and, most important, a Babe will take risks for the sake of truth. That's a skill April has yet to learn.

April and Randy have a pretty good sex life, but April has one big complaint: Randy is very quiet in bed. She still fantasizes about her ex-lover, Gary, who could keep up a sexy monologue that would send her to the moon. Sometimes Gary described his most out-there fantasies, sometimes he waxed poetic over April's porcelain skin or the feel of her grip on his penis, and sometimes he'd threaten to "make her" do really nasty things! Gary and April loved to play on an imaginative, vocal edge. In fact, once or twice April even had an orgasm from his words alone.

Trouble is, April can't bring herself to tell Randy what she wants to hear. She's afraid he'll think she's weird, afraid he'll say no, afraid he'll fail to measure up to Gary. If she doesn't ask, she can't be disappointed, shamed, or hurt—can she?

Actually, April's withholding is a huge barrier to closeness with Randy, and it's representative of all the other little withholdings she perpetuates in her relationship, all the other intimate expressions that she keeps in check out of fear of being revealed so nakedly. Eventually, all the withholdings that keep April from being authentic with Randy will eat away at the relationship like termites beneath a fresh layer of house paint. April will have to learn to take greater risks in the name of honesty before she can call herself a Babe.

Developing Authenticity

Our authentic self is who we are when unconcerned with judgment, with fitting in, with presenting an image that draws others. Your authentic self is ever-evolving, but it can remain shrouded in self-delusion if you are not willing to peer beneath your comforting surface.

Expressing authenticity can occur only after you decide you want to know yourself. Many people skip over this important step as they near adulthood, and instead follow the lead of their peers or give in to pressure from their families. If all your friends are getting married, you might think that marriage is the answer for you and tie up with the first willing candidate. If everyone around you is partying and slacking, you might follow the crowd, even if the nightlife feels empty. If your pals are all going on to grad school and you're feeling pressure from your family to sit for the LSAT, you might do what's expected without stopping to question what your choices mean—what they say about who you are. It's far easier to be a sheep than to be authentic—but Babes are NOT sheep!

One of the best shows on television, for many reasons, is *Buffy the Vampire Slayer*. One of the reasons is that amidst all the manic mayhem, the characters keep evolving, keep trying to tap into the best parts of themselves, and recreate themselves. Season after season, even vampires seek their reflection and search for their souls. It's just this sort of endless self-interrogation that entices your authentic self out into the open and commands growth.

BABE BOOSTER

Spend an hour at a large newsstand and take note of whatever really appeals to you or piques your interest. You may be surprised to find that it's time to upgrade your subscriptions according to your true desires.

The Puzzle of Sexual Authenticity

For each of us, sorting out who we are as sexual beings, deep down, unfettered by society's repressive rules, is a formidable task—but a Babe is up to it!

The most common question I receive from readers of my advice columns or hear from clients is, "I have these desires...am I normal?" Everybody carries the shame that comes with having a thought, a hunger, a passion that they fear is "abnormal." Heaven forbid we should savor the uniqueness in our eroticism!

Of all the soft- and hard-core lessons about sex that come our way as we are growing up, the insidious indoctrination in shame is perhaps the most stifling. Women are taught to be alluring and sexy, yet we are also taught to pair the experience of actual sexual desire with guilt, shame, and self-sacrifice. A Babe is able to sift through all these contradictory messages and see the truth—the only real shame is in devaluing the treasure of her sexuality, in failing to accept erotic freedom with a sense of sweaty, playful, liberating pride.

A Babe is always on the lookout for the shifty inner critic's voice that masks her own truths and mimics sexual edicts that originate outside herself. A Babe learns to pluck that critic's voice right out of her head, or she maintains a stock of gags in various colors and sizes for those times when it's stuck there, and just too insistently mouthy to contend with nicely!

A Babe checks in with her authentic self before making sexual choices. Even then, she might make mistakes, but when she does, she knows that she has seized upon a useful lesson. She realizes that there is no such thing as guaranteed emotionally safe sex or safe living, because life is composed of calculated risks and the only way to grow is to bring it on!

B IS FOR BOLDNESS
A Babe is excited by the unfamiliar. She feels alive and expansive when she dares to:

- ask a guy for a date, even though she thinks he's a little out of her league. (But then, being a Babe transcends leagues!);
- walk alone into a sex shop to buy a violet silicone dildo;
- say, "I love you" first;
- say, "It feels wonderful when you...." or "I'd love it if you would...." to let her lover know what she likes—both in or out of bed;
- greet her lover's idea for a sexy new antic with automatic enthusiasm, without looking for ways to poke holes in it first. If it's a real bust, "never again in this lifetime!" can come later;
- make a list of all the scary things she fantasizes doing, from jumping out of an airplane to jumping into a threesome, and then tick them off one by one as she unabashedly does what she has never done before!

In a Babe's life, boldness and authenticity function like sidekicks, backing each other up. Put another way, we could say that authenticity is the stone and boldness is the slingshot. Boldness propels your authentic self in a speeding arc out into the world.

A budding Babe need only access the tiniest kernel of boldness to discover how it thrives on being activated. You needn't make drastic leaps if you've been on the shy side until now—baby steps will do. If you take one risk—perhaps by practicing a couple of the exercises later in this book, or by slightly altering you *modus operandi* in one important relationship—as good things come of it (and they usually do!) you'll find yourself getting high on your success. Every time you reach beyond your comfort zone to make another small but meaningful change, feelings of pride and excitement will invigorate you. Then, when the next opportunity to stretch yourself crops up, you'll be more motivated to take yet another chance. Each time you venture forward bravely again, your boldness reserves will swell. Being bold is an investment in yourself that pays multiple dividends.

> **BABE BOOSTER**
> *You don't need to know everything or be a control freak to exude an air of confidence. It just takes practice, practice, practice!*

Back in the seventies and eighties, "assertiveness" was a catchword among feminists. Dozens of books and articles on becoming assertive appeared; classes and assertiveness trainings sprouted across the nation along with frozen yogurt shops and tanning parlors, and a raft of political discussions about the difference between being assertive and aggressive ensued. It was cool for a woman to be assertive—but aggressive, oh dear, no. That implied being much too...well...*bold* for the era. Today we don't want to draw those arbitrary limits. We can choose between gentle assertion and kick-ass aggression—though it's best to develop discernment before going the kick-ass route. Ripping open your boyfriend's shirt and clamping your mouth on his perky nipple is certainly aggressive, but do you really think he'd mind? Being bold means being willing to stake your claim and take your chances, even knowing that no matter how well chosen your bold moments, you won't always get the response you're hoping for. Nobody is going to score one hundred percent, but a Babe dusts herself off, files away her lesson, and keeps getting bolder.

For the record, being bold is not to be confused with being insensitive, boorish, or abrasive. We all know women who, in the name of assertion, step on other's toes with no regard for their feelings or needs. Being demanding and behaving rudely is not an emboldened Babe's style. I'm no

Miss Manners, and certainly no fuddy-duddy, but I do believe that even the boldest of Babes acts with plain-as-pudding politeness more often than not. Kindness and boldness are anything but mutually exclusive.

E IS FOR EROTICISM

I think I've spent half my adult life in restaurants. It's where I do most of my socializing, so it's also where I tend to do a great deal of my people-watching. Granted, it gives me a rather skewed view of the world. There aren't a lot of children in my world, or much cigarette smoke, but there is something about watching people in restaurants that's as close to watching them in their bedrooms as one can get. I see couples who eat together coldly, disengaged, and I often wonder if they sample each other's bodies just as perfunctorily when they make love. There are couples who flirt across a table with only their eyes, spilling a thousand secrets with every glance. There are women who extend their sexuality with every unself-conscious touch of their partner's hand, every easy giggle, every sinuous crossing of one leg over the other.

> **BABE BOOSTER**
>
> *Do one small thing each day (anything from wearing lipstick to wearing a garter) that makes you feel like a sex goddess.*

In thinking about women who convey eroticism without being overtly sexual, I recall one of my birthday dinners a few years ago. At the table beside my boyfriend and I were two men and a woman. The woman was attractive without being especially pretty, but she did have a rather ideal body that she moved in space with such grace and languorous comfort that her dinner companions were riveted—and so were we. Both my honey and I found ourselves glancing her way often, and when she stood up to go to the ladies' room we both followed her undulating movements with our eyes. We turned to each other and smiled appreciatively. "You'd love to take her home with us, wouldn't you?" I said. He laughed, "I think *you'd* like that." "I might," I teased and leaned into him to touch his thigh and kiss him on the mouth before we both returned to our gnocchi in gorgonzola sauce.

The woman in the restaurant was so connected to her abundant sexuality, that without doing anything improper she captured our attention and stimulated our juiciest thoughts. Because I, too, am quite firmly grounded in my sexuality, it was fun to use her presence as an invitation to my partner to take a brief, carefree excursion into fantasy.

We often speak of women or men being "in their power." It's a phrase that describes the sense of confidence, self-assurance, and effectiveness that some people exude quite naturally. People who stand in their power needn't be domineering or directive. They reek of power in the way they look straight into your eyes, shake hands firmly, and ask a question with the quiet authority of their interest. Likewise, a woman who stands in her eroticism carries herself with sensual pride. She doesn't have to dress in clingy clothing or wear a size four, though she might. She's so comfortable with her sexuality that she can't avoid exuding it any more than she could avoid exuding humor or friendliness, if those traits defined her. A Babe revels in the high fire of her eroticism and urges other women to do the same. Claiming your eroticism is an act of resolve that innervates every dimension of your life, not just the sexual. Writers on the subject of female sexuality often limit their discussions to sensual pleasure, orgasm, and the burning feeling we all seek in intimate relationships. That's good stuff, but there's a bigger picture.

Our authentic eroticism—the deep, scorched-earth layer of heat that glows like a single white-hot coal at the very center of the earth—is a source of explosive creative energy. It is the base "wanting" that galvanizes our assertions of competence and control. *Erotic power is personal, sovereign power. It is the nitroglycerine behind creative expression and resolute action. When you suppress any part of your eroticism, you suppress nothing short of your full aliveness.*

Babe, we are not foolin' around here!

When you are grounded in your sexual splendor, your every romantic relationship, whether it's serious or casual, reflects this solid, respectful sense of yourself as a loving, desiring being. Your eroticism is a gift to yourself which you express as you choose.

It's just about that simple.

Toward Ecstasy

Balance, authenticity, boldness, and eroticism: These are a Babe's vital possessions, the keys to reinventing yourself as the sexually adventurous woman you yearn to be. In the course of developing these qualities, you'll undertake a process corresponding to the two sections of this book:

Part I: Overcoming Romantic Obsessions

Part II: Cultivating Ecstasy: Having the Sex Life You Deserve

Here in Part I, Overcoming Romantic Obsessions, we'll explore obsessive romances and their intoxicating but often demoralizing chemistry. You'll see how you might have developed a yen for love affairs that replicate the enmeshed intimacy you grew up with. You'll meet women a lot like yourself who have exchanged their painful love affairs for joyous, rewarding relationships, and you'll learn how to peel away the thick layers of your personal history to reveal a rich capacity for empowered love and desire.

In Part II, Cultivating Ecstasy: Having the Sex Life You Deserve, you'll see why obsessive relationship styles are hardly the only impediments to having the erotic life you crave. We'll touch upon the myriad ways our culture attempts to stunt and repress women's powerful sexuality. I'll show you how you can free yourself from this unfortunate legacy and open yourself to ecstasy. We'll concentrate on loosening your erotic imagination, mining your deepest desires, giving reign to your fantasies, and discovering your body's sweet spots. Finally, you'll learn the ten unbeatable Babe's Rules (nothing like those *other* rules you've heard about!) for enjoying daring erotic exploits and turning sexually stagnant relationships into sources of exuberant pleasure.

You have much to look forward to, so let's begin.

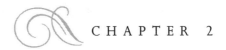

CHAPTER 2

The Roots of Romantic Obsession

Stop obsessing

R OMANTIC OBSESSION is part of our everyday language of love. Obsession, as I speak of it here, is a preoccupation with wild love, love gone wrong, or love just plain gone. In obsession, we may feel overtaken by a new love or overwhelmed by a longstanding troubled relationship.

Take Jeri, for example, whose story you'll hear shortly. During her relationship with Ray, she experienced ecstatic moments that made her come alive, punctuated by roiling conflict that left her in a state of raw anxiety. Ray was never far from her thoughts and it was hard for her to spend an evening with friends without giving in to the need to speak at length about her topsy-turvy love affair. Jeri's saga was almost as disturbing to her loved ones as it was to her, lost in the dizzying swirl of it. Yet, because tales like Jeri's are so common and rarely end in tragedy, I refer to them as the "soft obsessions."

There are other, more dangerous forms of obsessive love that are "hard obsessions." These deeply pathological scenarios are familiar to us, too—hopefully only because tabloid television and movies-of-the-week bring them into our homes. We hear of obsessed *erotomaniacs* stalking celebrities. We hear of ex-partners or rejected suitors who threaten, methodically intimidate, and sometimes do violence in their driven, consuming need to control the object of their so-called love.

You won't read tales of these hard obsessions here. Relationships that end in heartache, not homicide, are the stuff of most of our lives, and thus the stuff of this book.

Are You Obsessed?

When caught up in romantic obsessions, we tend to speak and think in characteristic ways. In making a dead-honest assessment of your own romances, answer the questions below and then count the number of yes answers.

Do you ever think or say:
- I can't live without him.
- I can't stop thinking about him.
- Each time he rejects me it just makes me more determined to show him how right I am for him.
- I've never been so crazy about anyone else before.
- Why can't he see that we're soul mates?
- I'll be okay when I can make him realize _____.
- I would do anything if he would only _____.
- If I only had a second chance I'd do it right this time.
- Nobody every loved me like this before—and no one ever will again.
- Nobody ever loved him like this before—and no one ever will again.
- I hate the way he makes me feel!

Scoring: If you answered yes to between three and five statements, you're teetering on the brink of obsession. If you answered yes to six or more, you're obsessed.

Profile of Obsession

Obsessed lovers tend to behave in characteristic ways, too. They often go to enormous lengths to exert subtle or direct control over their partners—even when they feel utterly out of control of themselves. In thinking about your relationships, count your yes responses to the following:
- I've called and hung up just to hear his voice.
- I drive by his house on purpose just to see whether he's home.
- I go out of my way to be where I know I can catch sight of him.
- I purposely try to make him jealous.
- I buy him gifts, write him poetry, and send cards to get his attention.

• I often zone out during conversations or meetings, ruminating over what to do about him.
• I go to great lengths to get him to change.
• I'm happy when he does what I need, and in despair when he fails me.
• My friends are beginning to get annoyed with the degree to which I talk about him.
• I've screamed terrible, accusatory things at him.
• I've fantasized about taking revenge on him for hurting me.
• I've slapped, hit, or pushed him, or he has been physically aggressive with me.
• I've harmed myself out of frustration or rejection.

Scoring: If you answered yes to more than three questions, or to only one of the last two items, you've entered the danger zone.

If you answered yes to six or more, you're in meltdown. (TAKE NOTE: If you answered yes to either of the last two items and you're not already in counseling, I urge you to talk with a therapist. Call your doctor or a close friend who can refer you to a counselor right away.)

Now, let's take a closer look at what these precarious attachments are all about. In obsessive relationships, five key qualities dominate. Think about your obsessive romances and consider which of the following characteristics are present. You'll usually find two or more of these in tandem. As more of them appear, the obsessive quality of the relationship escalates:

1. Unsatisfied emotional longings coupled with sustained sexual hunger.
2. A cycle of painful separations or conflicts alternating with joyous reconnections.
3. An insatiable appetite for more, more, more from the lover, and a tendency to turn somersaults to gain attention, commitment, or expressions of love.
4. Sabotage or near-sabotage of other life goals, including careers, friendships, education, and financial security.
5. Absence of efforts to step back from the relationship, gain perspective, and make choices based on reality, not on a fantasy of what might be, could be, or ought to be.

Reading this list of features in black and white, it seems inconceivable that we could accept these as attributes of "true love." Yet, since most of us were practically weaned on fictional depictions of love as obsession, it's not so surprising. If we rely on the stuff of movies and novels as our guide to relationships, we learn that we won't get the intoxicating sex life we deserve by *overcoming* obsessions. Instead, we'll get it by seeking out mind-melting affairs with lovers who wrest shrieking climaxes from us with one hand while ripping our hearts out with the other! If the stories we're told can be trusted, these are the relationships we should be *collecting*, not resisting. But, on-screen dramas make little distinction between healthy passions and unbalanced, scarring loves. Society and the broader media set us up for romantic failure by peddling fairy tales and *Sex in the City*–style plotlines that rarely exist in real life. When we stumble upon a relationship that begins with a bang, we imagine that we've been touched by destiny and cling stubbornly to the fiction that our new love is "The One," even as unmistakable signs to the contrary begin to stack up.

BABE BOOSTER

It's fine to watch Sex in the City *and relish in the gals' glamorous NYC romps—just don't make their sexcapades a compass for your intimate relationships.*

Finding My Babe

There was a period in my life when I would have hid under the bed to avoid disclosing my score on the Obsessive Love Quiz! I bought so thoroughly into a mythology that placed drama at the heart of passion, that even after I wised up and consciously let go of the myth, I was still vulnerable to it's ingrained message. Thankfully, time is a great healer, and an even better teacher. I found that being preoccupied by a relationship is the path neither to happiness nor to sexual ecstasy.

That lesson occurred quite a few years ago when I became embroiled in a thrilling, brain-rattling romance that turned into a sorry tale of devastation and loss. When the affair ended, I was certain that a corner of my heart had frozen over—that I'd forever be a beige, bland version of my once primary-hued self.

Of course, I was quite wrong. That was me, pre-Babe. I had no conception of the erotic aliveness, the sexual power, the deep love I was yet to encounter. In the absence of romantic obsession, the most remarkable possibilities lay before me, but like many women who can barely put one foot in front of the other after such a complex relationship collapses, the concept of future happiness was impossible to comprehend.

My relationship with Eddie began after a very difficult period in my life. I actually thought I was handling everything quite well, but I was far more vulnerable than I knew. He began weaving his spell the moment we met: "I fell in love with you the second I set eyes on you," he confided barely an hour into our first conversation. I laughed off his ridiculous claim, but I was smitten, too, by his dark good looks and exceptional charm.

Eddie and I never dated casually. From the beginning we attached to one another as if we'd known each other for a lifetime. Yet, we were so different. During our first weeks together we'd lie on our backs for hours, heads meeting upon a single pillow, weaving the stories of our lives into a shared diary. I was a hard-core city girl, and Eddie had grown up on a cattle ranch in a world glutted with macho pride and rough-hewn pain. The harshest part of his life was revealed much later on, after we'd been together for nearly a year. By that time, the smooth fabric of our early months had frayed, giving way to a more tumultuous love.

When Eddie was eight, he and his parents and two brothers were returning home from the movies. The winter day was bitter, the country roads were icy, and his father drove the family Buick into a tree. Eddie and his mother were propelled from the wreck into a powdery drift and landed side by side like snow angels. Eddie remembers lying in the cold twilight staring at his mother's hushed and still form, knowing instinctively that she was dead.

The morning of the crash, Eddie told me, his mother had punished him for some long-forgotten fault. Eddie, humiliated, had raved at her, "I hate you. I wish you were dead!"

A little later she was.

Some months following these revelations, Eddie told me that he had never loved a woman as much as he loved me—except, that is, for his mother. And because he loved me, he could confess the truth about his mother's death, about how he felt his rage had killed her, and how he had never recovered from her loss. Hearing this, my stomach clenched in fear, momentarily snapping me out of my obsessive cloud, but in the end, I shoved my body's warning aside and held him close.

Not long afterward, Eddie had surgery to repair an injured knee. I cared for him when he returned home from the hospital. He was edgy and more volatile than usual but I thought little of it—pain can do that to a person. Then one night, he picked a fight with me and foolishly I took the bait. We were both angry, yelling, and out of nowhere he sprung at me. I never saw it coming. When I managed to get free, I fled the house and two days later moved out. I know I made the right decision to leave, but I felt like the walking dead, staring for hours at blank walls.

Eddie was consumed by self-recrimination and blame. "I love you, I can't imagine life without you. Come back and let me prove it...please." And then, in puzzlement, "I don't know why you had to make me so angry." He said this on the telephone, his voice reverberating in the air between us.

"I DON'T KNOW WHY YOU HAD TO MAKE ME SO ANGRY."

I felt as if I were careening backward down a time tunnel. In that instant, I knew I had heard those words before—not from Eddie, but from my own mother.

My mother's anger, always vocal, would give way to days of unbroken silence. Eventually, her stony resolve would crumble and she'd wrap her arms around me. "I love you so much...you're my first baby...why do you have to make me so angry?" She, too, was truly puzzled, as though she were the child and I the grown-up whose acts were simply incomprehensible—instead of the other way around.

HISTORY LESSONS

Eddie and I, lost in a recapitulation of our pasts, were the poster couple for romantic obsession. Obsessive love is nothing if not a historical web in which childhood dramas converge and tangle in the adult present. Thankfully, I finally understood the original draw to Eddie, the remarkable interweaving of our lives.

Tempestuous relationships like the one I just described are an emotional and sexual thrill ride, exhilarating in a way one imagines will never be matched in the same lifetime. But the commotion inevitably gives way to exhaustion, and we lose bits and pieces of our self along the way.

The replication of early relationships is one of the reasons that romantic obsessions cannot give us the sex life we deserve, why they are obstacles to power and to love that is healthy and freely chosen—no matter how intensely passionate they *seem* to be. We deserve sex lives that enhance our capacities for deep connection *in the present*, for respect and caring between lovers. We deserve sex lives that give us a rush because our experiences are anchored in a sense of authenticity—we like who we are when we're with our partner, and we like who *he* is. As tempting as obsessive romances may be, we can do so much better than merely reliving our complex early attachments and elevating them to the status of myth.

Babes and Boundaries

A Babe can live without lash-thickening mascara, a laser-whitened smile, or a firm C-cup. But a woman can't really call herself a Babe until she develops distinct, firm boundaries. Let's take a closer look at what boundaries are all about.

Imagine drawing a picture of yourself with red chalk on a blackboard—a simple picture, just outlines. The red lines that define your figure and separate it from the surrounding space are, literally, your boundaries. Now, imagine erasing the red chalk on just the right side of your image. Do you see how you suddenly bleed into the blackboard or how the blackness seeps into you? On the left side of the figure the red boundary defining you is clear, but on the right side you can't see where you end and the slate begins. You and everything around you are one.

> **BABE BOOSTER**
>
> *Don't deny where you came from—you can learn lots from casting a truthful eye on your past—but don't dwell in it, either. Living in the NOW is where it's at.*

When your emotional red lines are sketchy and easily erased, it's hard to know where you end and others begin, or where your needs begin and others' end. You have trouble standing up for yourself—strong and separate—secure in who you are and what you feel.

A loss of distinct boundaries occurred in my relationship with Eddie. Similarly, Jeri's relationship with Ray is the story of two people whose boundaries became so hazy that their identities practically adhered to one another. As often happens, Jeri didn't know that she had lost touch with herself until a crisis occurred—and she was forced to redraw her red outlines.

THE ROLLERCOASTER RIDE

With his lean, brooding good looks and his unusual style of rhyme, Ray caught Jeri's attention in a songwriting class. Her attraction peaked when Ray invited her to an open-mike reading at a local coffeehouse. There, his fluid verse and the presence of his fawning ex-girlfriend, a gorgeous lingerie model whom Ray nearly ignored in favor of Jeri, bathed him in a sexy glow. From that night on, Jeri's relationship with Ray became the center of her world.

"Being with Ray was like jumping into a kaleidoscope and being spun around," Jeri told me later when the love affair had fallen apart and she entered therapy. "I stayed with Ray partly because I'd never felt so sensually alive and I was afraid I'd never find that feeling again," Jeri confessed. "It was a chemical thing—the timbre of his voice, the scent of his skin, the way our bodies locked together—all of it made his grasp on me tighter than I'd ever imagined any could be."

Jeri's recognition of why she was drawn to Ray illustrates how lovers always become one another's teachers. Even in painful relationships, our lovers help us confront the sides of ourselves that we don't acknowledge. When a woman like Jeri is out of touch with her eroticism, she may become attached to a man who brings out the juicy, sexually abandoned part of herself. As long as she imagines that her capacity for passion comes from him, she'll believe she needs him in order to feel fully alive—and she may put up with a lot of misery to hang onto that passion. In the beginning, the misery is never anticipated. Only later, after she's hooked, does the pain settle in and become an almost accepted part of the thrill.

Jeri and Ray began dating right after the open-mike event, and within a month they had moved in together. At first, Jeri wasn't so sure that living together was a great idea. Ray wasn't working full-time and she feared that she'd be stuck making the rent while he waited for a break as a spoken-word artist. Jeri's work as a financial executive in the record industry fed her comfortable lifestyle, but music and poetry fed her soul. Briefly, Jeri wondered whether her financial security and contacts in the recording industry were more of a lure for Ray than true love, but she reminded herself that with his talent and attractiveness he could have anyone—why choose her unless she was really special?

Once they began living together, Jeri saw that Ray was temperamental, demanding, and irresponsible. His moods were alternately exuberant and black, yet, in a fit of creative genius, Jeri found him irresistible. "He'd read his work to me, and I'd be lost in the amazing interplay of words and the crooning silkiness of his voice. We usually made love afterward. It was a wild aphrodisiac."

The more Ray's writing compelled Jeri, the less attention her own art received. "I couldn't compare my talent to Ray's," said Jeri. "He was sterling, and I was brass. Besides, when I wasn't working, I wanted to spend as much time with him as I could, and chaining myself to the computer to write chintzy verse didn't make sense anymore."

Right there, at the turning point where Jeri determined that Ray's work held more value than her own, her boundaries collapsed. Right there, Jeri merged with Ray so completely that the relationship could only grow more obsessive as time wore on. Jeri's boundaries had become too permeable—riddled with big holes where her precious self squished out and Ray's identity rushed in. She lost her separateness, allowing Ray to flood her with his feelings until they almost replaced her own.

The boundaries that we need in order to preserve, protect, defend, and illuminate us are like our psychic skins. Your self-boundaries are not nearly as perceptible as the visible wrapping of your body, your physical boundaries, but you can recognize the invisible psychic essence that holds you together by virtue of the way you relate to others. You can feel the intactness of your boundaries when you act on strong principles instead of impulse—when you can let your lover bleed as necessary without becoming his tourniquet. While it's true that when you are subjected to stress in a relationship you run a greater risk of forgetting yourself and relinquishing your boundaries, it's also true that under duress you have the opportunity to affirm them. Babes always get to choose.

Jeri chose to merge with Ray—to let Ray's emotions and needs seep into spaces where hers belonged and nullify them. When Ray exploded with impatience or criticism, Jeri took it upon herself to soothe him, tell him how much he meant to her, help guide him over each rough spot— even when Ray's fault-finding extended to her. When Ray was feeling good, when his energy spiraled, she flew on his joy, and when his sexual needs dominated, the two made love three, even four times a day. Jeri lived breathlessly on the edge because Ray did, while he reaped the benefits of having her as his stable, doting ally.

About eight months into their relationship, Ray's behavior grew even more erratic. The night he flew into a true rage, Jeri told him to leave. By doing this she reaffirmed one boundary, but she had lost touch with her ability to do so in the ways that really counted, day to day.

Predictably, in Ray's absence, she thought of him constantly. She drove by the house where he was staying, and she phoned him and hung up when he answered because she didn't know what to say. She spoke of him to her friends until they were sick of his name. She cried herself to sleep. She couldn't bring herself to ask him to come back, yet she couldn't stand the distance. She finally made a deal with herself—if he begged to come home, she'd give in, and when he appeared at the front door spewing apologizes, asking forgiveness, she let him in.

THE SEXUAL FALLOUT

In emotionally and sexually charged love affairs like Jeri and Ray's, where partners depend on each other for substance and form, desire becomes vaporous. It's difficult to know whose desire is being acted upon at any given moment. Jeri couldn't have told you whether she made love out of her own yearning or whether Ray's desire *for* her existed as her experience of her own desire. When she melted with him into a single, lustful expanse, there was no separating her hunger from his. For that reason, despite the sizzling quality of the affair, Jeri's relationship with Ray denied her the full power of her sexuality.

Whenever we are in a relationship where boundaries are hazy, eroticism seems to rise up out of our submergence in our lover, perpetuating the falsehood that the sexual hunger is not a part of me but a manifestations of *he*, or at best, *we*. We fear that if we lose the love affair, we lose all the erotic aliveness pent up within it, too. Only when we learn that the sexual magic we feel comes from within us—it doesn't belong to him—can we make healthy decisions about our current partner, or any other.

The Magic Mirror

When we fall into the abyss of love, we feel as if our most private, mythic fantasy has sprung to life. Finally, someone mirrors us perfectly, and we are rescued for a moment from all our self-doubt, fear, and isolation. Our body's rhythms come alive, for in the eyes of our lover we are desirable, special. We desperately need our lover to remain that magic mirror for us, so the moment we recognize our twin soul in him, we feel not only the joy of discovery, but also the fear of impending loss. A primal terror slips stealthily into place: "Oh my God, what if he goes away?" Meanwhile, the constancy of our lover's touch, taste, and scent produces a neurochemical trance that binds us. In this heady state, lovemaking may become an experience of melting, like two pats of butter set in a scalding pan.

BABE BOOSTER

Don't stay with a guy just for the great sex. There's a virtual sea of men out there who will respect your boundaries and shake you to your core!

In obsession, our primitive survival instincts kick in. Holding onto *him* is holding onto our very being. At the precipice of obsession we might do anything—suffer any indignity—just to keep him close. The one and only thing we cannot do is simply let go.

EXTREME OBSESSION

Jeri's obsession took its next dramatic turn a week after Ray moved back into her house. Jeri came home early from a meeting and was shocked to discover Ray snorting lines of cocaine off her glass dining room table. Ray accused Jeri of spying on him, but Jeri had to wonder, did he really want to be discovered?

"He eventually broke down sobbing and confessed he'd been doing drugs on and off for years. That's why he had such mood swings, and that's why he was always broke," she told me. Jeri was irrationally relieved to know that the source of their problems was something concrete that could be remedied. If only Ray cleaned up, they could be the perfect couple. Trouble was, Ray had no money or insurance for drug rehab. But Jeri did.

"I did the most impulsive thing—I married him to get him on my company's insurance plan."

When Ray left rehab, Jeri dedicated herself to helping him get his career up and running. She believed that his inability to succeed in the music industry had been at the heart of his drug use and she didn't want him to relapse. She called in favors, set up auditions and saw to it that Ray's talents were properly showcased. She did everything she should have and could have been doing to advance her own music career, but she had given up her belief in herself and put all of her faith in Ray instead.

The night Ray told her that he had inked a record deal with a small label Jeri was ecstatic. "I took him out to an expensive restaurant to celebrate. We drank champagne until we could barely walk, we fantasized about what life would be like when he was a star and I was his manager. And then, suddenly, the whole evening turned to ashes. Ray accused me of being jealous, of resenting all I'd done for him because I'd given up my own songwriting aspirations. No matter how much I reassured him, he grew angrier—as if it were my fault that he felt guilty about what I'd done. He kept talking crazy and there was no pacifying him. How could something so exciting turn into something so ugly?"

Even in his overwrought state, Ray had unveiled a truth that Jeri had been unwilling to face: *Her focus on him had usurped her love for herself!*

When Jeri woke up the next morning, it was with the certainty that Ray was doing drugs again—she'd seen the signs and had denied them. When she confronted Ray, he blew up. How dare she accuse him after all he'd done for her!

"All you've done for me?" Jeri screamed shrilly, the absurdity crashing in on her.

A financial whiz, Jeri knew all about debits and credits. Suddenly, when she looked at the ledger of her relationship with Ray, she saw how it tilted in his favor. "That was the end for me," said Jeri, looking back on that day. "The decision to break off the relationship was gut-wrenching, but I felt so used, so hurt. Besides, it was necessary. He was on cocaine, and I was on a very powerful drug called Ray."

A Powerful Drug

The reasons women like Jeri become so intoxicated with their lovers are varied, but disastrous relationships have a dark root in common. Certainly, the constant fluctuation between emotional extremes makes a relationship most seductive and addictive. The relationship builds to a crescendo based on intermittent excitement. Once the relationship ends and the contact with the person is withdrawn, getting over the relationship is like leaching a toxin from your system. Yet, it is the weakness of our boundaries that gives these relationships their power in the first place. It's no wonder that most of us are susceptible to obsessive romances at various points in our lives. We grow up conditioned to merge. If you have been in an obsessive relationship, chances are you did not get solid lessons in boundary building at home. As much as your parents loved you and tried to do their best for you, they were probably unable to keep from overwhelming you with their emotional demands.

Children often become the looking glass through which Mom and Dad see themselves—the test of their competence, a source of validation. The reassuring distance that gives a child room to discover all the facets of herself is violated by parental neediness. Most kids don't develop sturdy boundaries because they don't grow up hearing the unwavering message: "You're okay just the way you are. And, you know what? I'm okay, too. You don't have to be afraid that something bad will happen if you don't take good care of me. I'm fearless enough to give you space and strong enough to set limits so you don't go too far."

Lack of clear boundary delineation by Mom and Dad is a covert form of emotional abandonment which seeds fears that stay with us as adults. When coupled with more overt abandonment—abuse, chronic illness, divorce, or death—the boundaries between others and ourselves grow even blurrier. One day, when we fall in love, the impact of these early bereavements becomes clear.

Jeri grew up in a family where a workplace accident had left her father partially physically disabled and emotionally unavailable. Her mother had shouldered the burden of support for Jeri and her three younger siblings, while Jeri, in turn, tried to fill her mother's every emotional need. Although she resented her mother's martyrdom, the irony is that she replicated this very quality in her relationship with Ray. Indeed, family history may have set Jeri heading down the path to obsessive love. She had handpicked Ray in a subconscious and fruitless effort to try to make the drama of her childhood come out all right this time.

Confusing Fusion with Love

Jeri and Ray not only lacked mutually sturdy boundaries, but their relationship also demonstrated the invariable consequence of having such hazy red lines. The result is *fusion*.

In Chapter 1, I talked about balance, about how a Babe needs to achieve balance between her drive to be close with others and her urge to develop an individual, self-contained *me*. In obsessive romances, the drive toward togetherness predominates, or more accurately, overpowers. When we lean too far toward attachment, we enter into fusion with our partner. Fusion is the glue that keeps a crazy, demanding love intact. The sense of being *one* that Jeri experienced is a sign of fusion. For Jeri, fusion manifested as the relentless hunger to be a part of Ray. For Ray, fusion took the form of alternations between clinging neediness and furious resentment.

BABE BOOSTER

Feistiness is fine, but in a volatile love situation, it's best to adopt a Zen attitude. Closed eyes and a few deep breaths should have you thinking clearly—instead of reacting rashly.

A hallmark of fused relationships is intense emotional *reactivity* to the anxiety that spikes and dips between loved ones. Reactivity is the opposite of thoughtful reflection. In our families, we grow up adapting to the shifting anxieties that float freely in our households. In homes governed by troubled marriages, addiction, or emotional instability, that anxiety and reactivity is often palpable even to outsiders.

As we are growing up, we struggle on our own to find a way to cope with family anxiety. Think back to your own childhood, where you might have learned that you could reduce your discomfort by stemming the tides of others' emotions—so you strained to please. Maybe you learned that by being hostile and accusatory you could lob the hot potato of anxiety into someone else's lap and set yourself free. Perhaps you felt too inept to manage assertively, so you took the blame for all the troubles in your home, or you grew depressed, or became compulsive about eating or watching television.

In my family, I learned that by being a fighter, I could defend against others' anxiety-driven bids for control. Remember the story about Eddie and I from earlier in this chapter? I made one big mistake at the outset of the argument that turned so treacherous—I let myself be lured into a fight in the first place. I felt threatened by Eddie's accusations, and my own boundaries dissolved. I reacted quickly out of my fusion with him, needing to make him wrong so that I could feel safe and strong. I did what I had learned to do as a child—act tough to hold others at bay.

You might have thought that by being willing to fight, I was asserting my boundaries. That's a mistake many of us make. I certainly made it! Had I been more thoughtful, I would have realized that there was no margin in fighting at that time, and even if I had wanted to address a problem with Eddie, I could have done it without raising the thermostat and making the scene more heated. An authentic assertion of boundaries is rarely inflammatory—spontaneous combustion is sheer reactivity. In most instances, we can protect our boundaries calmly while deescalating a tense situation rather than inciting a riot.

Fusion is very common, and dramatic reactivity to the anxieties produced by fusion is so ubiquitous that it might seem like there is no other way to exist in the world. Actually, there is—which brings us back to the topic of balance, balance being the first B in Babe.

Make It "All about Me"

In order to achieve a healthy balance between the togetherness urge and the draw to being an individual, we need to return to the *differentiation* concept I mentioned in Chapter 1. Differentiation is the ability to sustain a clear, defined sense of self in the face of opposition and anxiety. Another way of addressing differentiation is to think of it as implying *self-focus* rather than *other-focus*. Not only does the idea of being self-focused have a less clinical, more user-friendly ring, but it also makes the self our reference point, the pivot upon which all else turns. Instead of putting the emphasis on another person—which is what you do when you're romantically obsessed—the center of the world of responsibility is you.

In Chapter 3, we're going to look at how becoming self-focused is the antidote to romantic obsession. But for now, let's consider in more detail how the absence of self-focus turns exciting romances into all-consuming obsessive loves.

THERE'S A DISTINCTION TO BE MADE
Self-focus is not selfishness or self-indulgence. Self-focus is the ability to remain thoughtful and clear about your own beliefs, values, and needs even when your lover exerts pressure on you to relinquish them or you are tempted to give yourself away. Remaining self-focused is one hell of a tall order, yet it is the key to being balanced and anchored in your own truth.

When a Babe is self-focused she:
- doesn't need her lover's constant approval to feel good about herself;
- doesn't succumb to pressure to change her personality or beliefs;
- can remain emotionally available to her lover even when she disagrees with him or feels angry;
- doesn't let herself become a sponge for her lover's anxiety, and doesn't jump through hoops to try to soothe his discomfort;
- can deal with her lover's upset without flipping out, giving in, counter-attacking, or running for the hills;
- can say "no" in a loving way;
- doesn't hunger to be one with her lover, but strives to be part of an intimate, mutually compassionate two;
- can take time to reflect on problems rather than resort to the quick-fix of being either pleasing or combative;
- can refrain from over-pursuing when her lover distances;
- can refrain from self-defeating behaviors (such as drinking, overeating, verbally attacking, sending reams of e-mail) when her anxiety level is high.

Understanding what self-focus is *not* can also help shed light upon what it *is*. Adrienne's relationship with Tony illuminates self-focus by showing us its opposite—focus on the other. As you read Adrienne's story, think about what Adrienne might have done a little differently at every phase of her relationship if she had been dedicated to being self-focused instead of hopelessly fused with Tony. In the next chapter, you'll see how well you did in choosing alternatives.

The Ultimate Makeover

Adrienne met Tony when he began teaching yoga classes at her gym. She was new to yoga, and Tony made a point of giving her a lot of special attention. One day she bumped into him at the supermarket—in the organic food aisle. His basket was brimming with fresh fruits and whole grains, and there she was, laden with chips and sweets. Adrienne tried to shuttle her basket behind her so that Tony wouldn't have a chance to see her purchases. "I was so attracted to him, but I worried that he wouldn't be interested in a carb addict like me! I wanted to get out of there fast!"

> **BABE BOOSTER**
>
> *Don't pretend you like kung-fu movies to snare a guy if that's really not your speed—the charade will leave you empty. Instead, confess your love of classical music and see what happens.*

Adrienne's nervous attempt to vamoose must have intrigued Tony. "The more I seemed to want to leave, the more Tony tried to hold me there. I should have remembered that clue to his character later. Tony likes a challenge."

The next day, Tony was at her side minutes after she arrived for her workout.

"Dinner Saturday night?"

He fired the invitation like an order without even saying hello. Adrienne giggled hesitantly. "I won't take no for an answer!" Tony insisted. She barely nodded, her heart pounding as if she'd spent half an hour on the Stairmaster.

When Saturday rolled around, Tony took her to a vegetarian restaurant. "I was in the mood for a thick, juicy steak with fries, but I ate nut and rice casserole instead. It wasn't too bad, and I pretended I was used to eating that gunk."

Tony spoke enthusiastically of his studies in naturopathic medicine. He'd be completing school in a few months and would move into an internship and then private practice. He spoke of his spiritual path and his interest in Tantra. Adrienne didn't dare ask what Tantra was for fear of sounding dumb. "Mostly I was mesmerized by his blue eyes and dimples. He was definitely the cutest guy I'd ever dated, and so smart. I wanted to know more about what he knew and I just hoped that he wouldn't discover what a regular girl I was."

Adrienne wasn't "regular" for long. She spent the following days boning up on New Age topics and filling her bookshelves with titles she thought might interest Tony and ensure she wouldn't appear shallow if he happened by her place.

Her homework paid off. Before long she and Tony were an item, and Adrienne was fixing mushy vegetarian casseroles for her new sweetheart, gagging down the bullet-sized nutritional supplements he brought over, and even meditating. He became her private guru, and a demanding one at that. "If I was in a bad mood he'd say that my negative energy was toxifying his space and send me off to do some kind of aura cleansing!" Any other guy would have said, "You're pissing me off," but not Tony. He was always coming from a place of spiritual goodwill.

When Adrienne moved in with Tony, the requisite changes in her lifestyle multiplied. Her best friend, Angie, worried that Tony was working too hard to make her into a new person, but Adrienne insisted he had only her health and welfare at heart.

"Sex with Tony was something else!" Adrienne exclaimed. "I found out pretty quickly what Tantra was all about, and it was yummy! Deep breathing, staring into each other's eyes, long, slow penetration where Tony barely moved inside me. My orgasms lasted for what seemed like hours and coursed through my whole body. Let me tell you, the sex made all the hoops I had to jump through for Tony worthwhile. Except, well, there were times when I just wanted him to toss me on the bed and bang the daylights out of me until I screamed like a banshee. That never happened." I asked Adrienne if she had ever expressed her desire to Tony. "Oh, no," Adrienne gasped. "He would have thought I was some depraved animal!"

Tantra gave way to group exercises in drawing erotic energy out of the power of communion among a small cadre of spiritual seekers. "We explored everything from erotic massage to spiritual transformation using psychedelic mushrooms, but mostly we shared sacred sex to connect with the divine." At first, Adrienne was anxious about these "ceremonies"

(Tony corrected her sternly when she accidentally called them orgies). As he encouraged her to free her erotic spirit, she came to enjoy the adventures that meant so much to the man she adored. "I had one teeny problem, though," Adrienne confessed. Watching Tony drive other women into paroxysms of ecstasy rankled her, but she was too ashamed of her jealousy to tell Tony.

The tables soon turned. At Tony's urging, Adrienne reached out in a sexual way to other women in the group and felt a passion she hadn't suspected could be so strong toward them. Tony, always so sure of himself, grew threatened—but rather than admit his fear, he became more controlling and hypercritical of Adrienne. Suddenly it was her clothes and her way of speaking that he attempted to alter. Adrienne, who had been momentarily thrilled with her sexual evolution under Tony's guidance, now sank into an anguished depression, realizing that no matter what she did, no matter how she modified herself, she couldn't quite satisfy him. She felt hopeless, sometimes even worthless. Adrienne's friend, Angie, suggested she and Tony seek therapy.

"Tony said that I was the one who needed a therapist—he was doing his consciousness work on his own. So like a good girl I came to see you by myself," Adrienne told me during our first session. A few months later she commented, "Looking back I have to thank him. Therapy has virtually shaken me out of suspended animation and made me see how shattered my self-esteem was, how obsessed I was with pleasing him."

Soon she reached an inevitable crossroad. "We were walking down the street and he began to lecture me over something I'd said or done that didn't meet his high standards. I don't remember what it was because at that moment it stopped mattering. My body went cold and rigid. A bus pulled up at the corner. I had no idea where it was going but without saying a word I jogged ahead of him and hopped on it. He stood there, stupefied. I thought, that's the last time I'll ever let him make me feel so powerless!"

Adrienne and Tony's story doesn't end here. But let's pause for a moment and consider the beginning of her tale. Did you notice how Adrienne set the tone for her relationship with Tony at the very outset? In the grocery store, her shame over her eating habits blocked any authentic connection with Tony. Rather than engage from a place of power and pride, the real Adrienne hid. Ironically, her attractiveness to Tony came out of what he mistook for self-assurance, but it was really anxiety manifesting as an urge to flee.

If we pay attention, our very first encounters with a prospective lover often reveal important truths about ourselves. Adrienne might have seen that her low self-esteem, which gave sway to her wish to emulate Tony's way of life, had marred the prelude to her relationship and threatened its progression. Even though she didn't learn that lesson as early as she could have, her relationship with Tony eventually became her teacher, though not exactly in the way that Tony intended. In Chapter 3, you'll see how Adrienne and Tony managed to breathe a second wind into their love affair as Adrienne learned to honor herself, draw boundaries, and develop self-focus.

Like Adrienne, any woman can achieve the balance she needs as a Babe in love.

Overcoming Romantic Obsessions and Setting Yourself Free

Become your own center of attention

N OT LONG AGO my client Carla asked me whether it was possible, in healthy relationships, to experience the striking intensity that comes with obsessive love affairs. It was a good question. She had just come up for air after months of playing romantic Russian roulette with a man who was unpredictable and mostly unavailable, but when he was with her, the edges of her heart curled like a love letter set aflame. So it made sense that she had an interest in this particular question, and it makes sense that you might, too.

Pick a Card: Depth or Intensity?

Carla's relationship with Danny was all about emotional intensity, built on rotating episodes of excitement, hope, and despair. The relationship started casually and ended cavalierly, but not because Carla wanted it that way.

They met at the hospital where he was a staff physician and she was a resident. Danny had just separated from his wife of eight years, making him a poor relationship prospect. Carla realized this, but she was only looking for a little tension release herself.

With Danny she got release, all right! Sex was hot and kinky, and all went well for the first few months, until Carla began daydreaming about

Danny when she should have been concentrating on her patients. Then, out of nowhere, Danny stopped calling and Carla went into a tailspin.

Never one to stand on ceremony, Carla tracked Danny down in the hospital cafeteria; she marched up to him with the four little words that men universally dread on the tip of her tongue: We need to talk.

"Not now," Danny said, "I'm in a hurry."

"NOW," Carla said, placing her hand on his arm and steering him toward a nearby table. Her pitch was high and her voice was louder than anyone else's. A few people stared.

"You're avoiding me," Carla stated. "I want to know what happened."

"Nothing happened," Danny insisted. "We didn't have any commitments, I got busy, life goes on."

How could he be so cold? Carla thought, panicking. Tears welled up in her eyes. And why was she reacting so strongly? He was right, they had no commitments.

"Look," Danny offered, "let's have dinner on Friday. We can talk then. I'll come over to your place and we'll have some privacy, okay?" Carla felt as though reprieved from death row.

On Friday, Danny showed up with flowers and, before Carla could get them into a vase, Danny was tearing at her clothes. All was well again. But a week passed and Carla heard nothing more from Danny. She grew restless, sleepless, and anxious. Worse, she realized that as much as she had been trying to deny the truth, she had fallen in love with him.

Carla's relationship with Danny was not really about love at all, it was about the intensity of passion offered and withheld—of craving, being satisfied, and then left to crave again. But in her fog, she could only imagine that Danny felt as she did. Just coming out of a broken marriage, maybe he didn't want to rush things—she could understand that. She only needed some reassurance. If he would admit his feelings, *then* they could take their time.

Danny popped up again when he needed Carla. He'd call to see whether she was home and then appear at her door. Occasionally they went out on actual dates and Carla's heart soared, but usually they played bedroom games until they were exhausted, and then Danny took off. For a few days Carla would ride a cloud, until the pain of separation and the anxiety of not knowing when she'd see him again hit. And so continued Carla's crusade to make Danny accept what she already knew—they were right for each other.

With Carla more attached to Danny than ever, each round of distancing flung her further into despair, a despair alleviated by hope and excitement when he reappeared filled with ardor and lust.

The cycle might have gone on far longer than it did, but events forced a turn. When Carla's residency ended, she was offered two full-time positions, the best one being a three hours' drive away. When she told Danny about the offers, he encouraged her to take the better one.

"What about us?" she asked.

Danny said, "We've had a good run. Maybe it's time to move on."

Carla felt as though she'd been kicked in the teeth, yet she was still sufficiently in touch with reality to see that if this was his response, then it was indeed time to move on. She couldn't get what she needed from Danny and if she stayed nearby, her obsession with him would never abate.

A Question of Reality

What about Carla's original question: Can she get this kind of intensity in a healthy relationship?

First, let's understand that Carla's so-called relationship with Danny wasn't an intimate relationship at all—it was a sequence of lustful encounters with little of substance to hold them together. Carla confused fusion with love. To have the same kind of intensity, she'd need the same cycle of excitement alternating with despair, then alternating with hope over and over again. Of course there's a special intensity to such a cycle that a healthy love can't match! Without the despair, an edge is missing—an edge as sharp as a blade, honed by one lover's obsessive, unrequited attachment and the other's intermittent distance.

Carla and Danny's relationship lacked even the pretense of intimacy. One does not find genuine intimacy in a relationship based on occasional sex and emotional fusion—a cycle of excitement/hope/despair. In a relationship blooming with intimacy, we experience a quality missing from fused relationships—depth.

In relationships where two self-possessed, self-focused people relate intimately, they experience depth. In relationships where boundaries dissolve and lovers fuse, there is intensity.

Surely you can get some intensity from a healthy love, Carla insisted, desperate to hear a "yes." It frightened her to think that a healthy relationship had to be dull as a spoon.

And it's true—where there is intimacy and depth there are often moments when lovers do fuse, when boundaries melt away for a little while, and, yes, it does feel yummy. But when it's time to step back from that momentary merging and anchor within your distinct selves again, you can. When your boundaries are strong, and you feel connected to your partner through confidence in the intimacy you share, you acquire the ability to go to those fusion-like depths at will and leave them by choice. The intimacy is also deeper, because you are two, appreciating one another; two, reaching *out* to one another and embracing one another, rather than two burrowing *into* one another, aching to become one.

Carla wasn't ready for that kind of intimacy because she was still looking for fusion. It would take some time for her to grasp the meaning or the power of developing clear boundaries and balance—but she'd get there.

Let me reiterate one of the key points from the previous chapter: Overcoming romantic obsession demands shifting your focus from the object of your desire to yourself.

The remainder of this chapter is about learning to focus on yourself, hold your center, and achieve the balance between closeness and individuality that is at the heart of genuine intimacy and is the keynote to being a Babe.

Adrienne and Tony: Developing Self-Focus

I think it's time for a success story, don't you? Let's return to Adrienne and Tony, who we met in the previous chapter. Adrienne was our modern Eliza Doolittle and Tony was her New Age Professor Higgins.

When Adrienne first came to see me, her self-esteem was at an all-time low. Her relationship with Tony had been all about trying to mold herself into a shape he could admire because Adrienne didn't feel good about the shape she was already in. Even though she loved Tony, the relationship had become unhealthy for her, and though Tony didn't know it then, just as unhealthy for him. Think of it—why would a man make such a concerted effort to remodel a woman into someone who is a carbon copy of himself? Because facing differences, even the slightest opposition, threatened Tony and left him feeling helpless and insecure. Controlling women allowed him to avoid self-doubt and conferred the illusion of strength. If Tony were ever to achieve the enlightenment he believed he already had, he would need to wake up to this truth.

The day Adrienne figured out that she and Tony were actually quite similar—both scared, both longing for a complementary safe haven—the unexpected "Aha!" left her breathless. "This is the most freeing moment of my life," Adrienne cried out. "I feel like nothing Tony can do will ever diminish me again!"

Ha! If only!

TIME FOR A REALITY CHECK

Ah, what an exquisite feeling to connect with ourselves so fully and deeply that we think we're invulnerable to being knocked off balance— that we'll never feel small, never hunger for approval again! But just as a Babe has bad hair days, even the staunchest Babe has bad *self* days, when her reactions are triggered all over again. This is real life, I'm afraid, not some psychological fairy tale, and in real life, balance is more a matter of degree than an absolute. Much as I wish I could promise that once you become a Babe you'll never veer off balance, old stuff does kick in now and then. But when a Babe momentarily loses her grip on herself, she catches herself quickly. Instead of luxuriating in fusion, she feels like she's trying to swim through molasses and craves the ease of floating through the warm, clean water of self-possession. She has no other choice but to lift herself up by her bra straps and plant herself more firmly in her power, because that's what feels good—that's what feels true.

Making Over the Ultimate Makeover

Let's return to where we left Adrienne at the end of the previous chapter. She had just hopped a magical mystery bus in her dramatic escape from Tony's barrage of criticisms, leaving him standing on the sidewalk in shock. Within days, she moved in with her friend Angie, and no amount of pressure from Tony could induce her to return home—quite unusual for Adrienne, who was so accustomed to giving in to Tony. But notice how one minute Adrienne was sticking to Tony like glue, and the next she was ripping herself asunder, fleeing his side as though he were on fire. These extremes of closeness and distance, pursuit and detachment, are hallmarks of fused relationships. Each attempt at a shift in the existing dynamic becomes a stunningly dramatic demonstration of oppositional behavior. Adrienne felt as though she had to run for her life because she was still so attached to Tony that unless she left tire tracks as she screeched away, she risked never rising off the pavement.

Despite her sensational exit, at least she did get out of Dodge, which gave her some breathing room and a chance to regroup and think through her options. Score one for Adrienne. End of First Act.

Act Two of this relationship began when Tony urged Adrienne to let him accompany her to therapy. Surprise. Not only did Tony's capitulation astound Adrienne, but it also gave her hope. Yet she didn't entirely trust Tony's gesture, uncertain whether it was just a ploy to lure her back into their power-imbalanced dynamic. But what if Tony really *did* want to do some serious work on himself and the relationship? Trying to figure out what was real, what Tony intended, started to drive Adrienne a little batty.

How many hours have you spent with girlfriends agonizing over lovers' motives? If you could add up all those hours, how many extra months—even years—would you be able to tack back onto your life and make available for other pursuits? And what might you have accomplished in that time? Self-focus begins when you stop wasting your precious, irretrievable hours trying to assess other people's motives! I know it's tempting, and maybe you're thinking: She must be kidding; she's a psychologist for goodness sake! Isn't figuring people out what she *does?* Well, yes—and that's the trouble, sometimes. If the guy is my client, it's one matter, but if he's my boyfriend, I'm way out of line.

We women are so used to obsessive analysis in the interests of fiddling with and fixing our relationships that the very thought of stepping back a pace sends us reeling. If we don't spend our time figuring him out (or her, if our romance is with another woman), then how do we know what to *do* in our relationships? That's the point, Babe: What we do should never be predicated on the other person, but on ourselves.

When Adrienne let go of wondering what Tony was really up to, then and only then could she end her obsession, then and only then could she begin the long, slow process of building her self-esteem. Sure, Tony could come to therapy, but Adrienne's big shift came the day she realized that it mattered not a whit whether Tony was authentically on board or just going through the motions. Because nothing Tony did could change Adrienne's direction, which was all about being real with herself, real with the big stuff like why was she willing to let Tony, or anyone, belittle her? And real with the small stuff—like did she want to keep gulping down those bullet-sized vitamins Tony put on her plate every morning? Well yes, actually, she did. Lo and behold, she felt good taking those horse pills. Did she want to engage in more group sex ceremonies? No. She'd been there, done that, and if she was going to continue exploring her erotic interest in women, she'd like to do it one gal at a time. Did she want to hear Tony wax philosophical from his elitist pulpit about her need for enlightenment, her manner of speaking, her mode of dressing? Not anymore. Does that mean that if Tony were to comment on the aforementioned she'd be entitled to jump down his throat for DARING to tell her what to do! Uh, no. Remember how reactivity denotes fusion? If she wishes to remain self-focused, she'll need to take a few deep breaths and say, "Thanks for sharing your thoughts, honey. I might consider that." Or, "Interesting point of view, lambkins, but I see things differently." And then, without drowning in the anxiety of opposing Tony, remain faithful to her principles.

> **BABE BOOSTER**
> *Abandon the idea of who "wears the pants" in your relationship. The best unions are those where two parties can give and take, and where there's no upper hand.*

Adrienne was becoming clearer about what self-focus meant to her, but the big puzzle was: Could she continue on her path indefinitely? Could she hang on to herself in spite of what Tony—whose authoritative presentation was unlikely to change much—said, did, or expected? For Adrienne, that was the question of a lifetime, because even if she and Tony parted ways, she'd come up against the same issues in any other relationship. Her challenge was in being authentic, balanced, and bold.

Now, here's the good news: Adrienne and Tony are still together, working on their relationship, still seeing me every other week, and both of them are growing in fits and starts, learning how to appreciate being "two" as a couple, and "one" as honorable, self-respecting individuals. They've achieved a lot, no matter where their relationship ultimately takes them.

Blueprint for Obsession: The Sorry Six

Just in case you've never been in an obsessive romance and, after reading these stories envy those who have, here's a blueprint for striking one up. The following tactics are guaranteed to keep you focused on your partner, keep your emotions twirling and spinning, and ensure your relationship grows more dramatic every day.

Okay, I'm teasing about hoping you'll use these tactics to create an obsessive love, but not about the utility of the methods. We grow up using these approaches to fend off anxiety and continue using them in romantic relationships when we feel threatened by loss, shame, or lack of control. Yet, here's the irony: Instead of being salve for our psychic wounds, they are salt.

Let's look at our blueprint for obsession, comprised of the six most striking and common styles of reacting to anxiety. All six can sensationalize ordinary interactions so that they reach soap opera proportions, (He: "Good morning." She: "How can you say that to me after last night? You're so insensitive!"). And, most important, all six usually leave one or both partners feeling regretful or embarrassed. That's why I call them the Sorry Six. Yes, they are a sorry lot indeed.

After you've read a section about each one of the six, take a moment to close your eyes and recall a time when you used that reactive style under fire. You might discover that you employ just a few of these approaches, or that you've tried your hand at all six. Before you begin, find a clean notebook or designate a computer file as a journal. Each time you open your eyes after scanning for memories, make notes of your recollections. They'll be useful later.

PURSUIT

Obsessive relationships are built upon pursuit. Pursuit is all about moving toward our lover and attempting to provoke a desired response, or at least some response! We can pursue confrontationally, as Carla did when she cornered Danny in the cafeteria and said, "We have to talk." We can pursue coyly, becoming sweet and compliant to try to appease an angry lover or engage a distant one. We can pursue aggressively, by bombarding our lover with e-mail and phone calls to command his attention.

Pursuit may also take the form of demands for reassurance, for expressions of love and desire that can seem stifling to the target of pursuit. "You never tell me you love me!" is actually a form of pursuit, for behind your complaint is a bid for an emotional response, for attention, or for a shift in behavior. In any case, you're saying, "Gimme!"

Pursuit and distance become a kind of lovers tango—the dancers may shift roles as the intensity builds. The pursuer becomes the distancer when she simply tires of pursuing or gets what she wants after great effort. In some relationships, one partner nearly always pursues while the other remains distant, as was the case in Carla and Danny's affair. The distant partner's unavailability and the pursuing partner's insatiable need bind them.

Pursuers often play a head game I call "I can make him." Women besotted with married or otherwise unavailable men perfect this game as an art. They play with the idea that these statements will become reality:

- I can make him prefer me.
- I can make him think of me all the time.
- I can make him love me.
- I can make him want to be with me all the time.
- I can make him marry me.

The rumination so common among obsessive lovers is actually a form of "magical" pursuit. You're keeping your partner close, prevailing upon him with all your will. By talking to you lover in your head, replaying conversations, over and over, you may even begin to believe you can magnetize him and make him come to you, ready to offer his devotion.

DISTANCING

Where would a pursuer be without a distancer? If you are the distancer, then, when your lover pursues, you pull back. You stop calling, you avoid answering the phone, you take your good-natured time responding to his e-mail. When you're with him, you're colder, quieter, disinterested in sex and in whatever he has to say to you about almost anything, from his work life to the feelings that he's finally, desperately sharing. You begin withholding all the tiny perks that you've been sprinkling along the seductive path of your love affair.

Distancing can be a way of punishing a lover for having detached earlier, or it may be a way of fielding behavior that threatens to engulf you. Distancing can be a last ditch means of trying to gain some badly needed space when you feel suffocated. In obsessive relationships, distancing occurs dramatically and intensifies the emotionality of the situation. For instance, when Adrienne left Tony, her move packed a wallop because it was a turnabout from her usual behavior. In reaction, Tony gave his own panicked pirouette a go.

Breaking up and making up is a distancer-pursuer dance, replete with dips and spin.

Rarely do distancers do their work conscientiously, like suggesting taking a day or two to think things through, with the promise of getting together at a specified time to reconnect. Oh, no, that's far too logical, considerate and fair. Instead, in obsessive relationships the distancer usually yanks the plug, leaving the pursuer in a state of extreme agitation, their worst abandonment fear realized. Now the pursuer's impetus to rush forward heats up. Funny, isn't it, that the distancer isn't the least bit surprised.

INCITING CONFLICT

There's always fodder for conflict in relationships. Couples do need to duke out their disagreements from time to time, and if they can argue constructively, i.e., without ripping each other's character to shreds, or being contemptuous or defensive, a good fight can clear the air. However, in obsessive relationships, conflict may stand in for loving intimacy. During conflict, partners *feel*, even if what they are feeling is anger or hate. Fuming is better than apathy, isn't it?

Conflict can become a smokescreen that obscures lack of genuine commitment, even lack of love. In obsessive relationships, we often excuse conflict—attributing it to passion—especially where the sexual chemistry is strong. When we are high on our own fumes, a golden cloud hovers around our relationship, and it's difficult to shine a fog light into the haze. Should a glimmer of clarity poke through, if we don't like what we see forming in the distance, renewed conflict can thicken the fog and keep us blindly engaged.

In conflict-ridden relationships, peace reigns for predictable periods. If you can't make it more than a week or two without a fight, you may be provoking anger to avoid anxiety over an aspect of the relationship that's unfathomably scary—far scarier than whatever you appear to be fighting about. Yet, it's that unseen dimension of feeling that's screaming to be addressed.

Dueling lovers often play consistent roles. One condemns, the other defends. One blames, the other stonewalls or defends by counter-attacking. Each of these styles is a means of reacting to the anxiety that bubbles like lava beneath the crust of the relationship, and it is this anxiety, and the pain it produces, that is so rarely acknowledged or soothed during these collisions.

TRIANGLING

When anxiety between lovers becomes unbearable, we drag a third party into the mix to carry some of the weight. The extramarital affair is the classic triangle: "I can't deal with my spouse, so I'll shift my attention to someone new." But close friends and family members are also easily triangled into a troubled relationship, helping to spread the heat around.

Statements like these indicate a triangle is forming:
- "My mother thinks you're a cad!"
- "Even your best friend says you shouldn't have treated me that way."
- "I'm sick of your jealousy over my friendship with Bob. You're making too much out of nothing!"

When the source of your conflict with your lover is a third party, whether it's your mother, your child, his wife, even your pet, you are triangling. Complaining to your best friend about your relationship, even though you think you're justified in venting or legitimately seeking support, is still triangulation of a sort, especially if your friend is also your partner's friend. Yes, we all triangle now and then, but just because we do it, and just because the venting or the actual advice we receive does provide solace, doesn't mean that triangling is any less problematic or less likely to keep an obsessive loop going.

BLAMING

Who among us has never blamed our partner for the troubles in our relationship? Yet, blaming is the pinnacle of other-focused behavior. So long as you remain fixated on what he did, what he needs to change, his warped motives—Tarzan bad, Jane good!—you lose sight of your own role.

The other day I spoke with a dear friend whose relationship is fraught with conflict over her lover's fractious distancing. She had been blaming him and his remove for the problems between them. When she feels insecure and begs for validation, he huffs, puffs, and blows the relationship away, dropping back as far as he can without disappearing entirely. Then she had a profound realization: Since her insecurities predate anything the relationship either caused or can heal, she wondered what might happen if she were to stop begging and let the relationship play itself out, giving him no reason to run due to her stifling need for reassurance. I believe she is making strides by viewing herself as a key player in this dynamic instead of exclusively blaming her partner.

Blaming need not even make sense to work as an escalation tactic. One of the most inane yet true-to-life blame scenes on film is depicted in *Your Friends and Neighbors*. Here, a misogynistic single gynecologist, who uses sex as revenge against women, lambastes his lover for bleeding all over his white, 380-thread-count Egyptian cotton sheets. As she huddles behind a locked bathroom door, he screams: "You are NOT a nice woman! I mean who in the FUCK just gets their period all of a sudden? It just doesn't HAPPEN—and it's HAPPENED all over my bedding. You knew that—and you're TWISTED to PLAN this!" The same film depicts other Sorry Six strategies with equally striking accuracy and frightening humor. I highly recommend the film.

VICTIMIZATION

As long as you see yourself as your lover's victim, you can't acknowledge the degree to which you made the relationship possible as it is, or why you made your particular choices each step of the way. Victims are likely to resort to blaming ("Look what you did to my sheets!") or pursuing ("Don't leave me like this!"). Filled with victim-rage, they may also become perpetrators of self-righteous, venomously indignant attacks. The how-dare-you attitude that on the surface sounds so tough comes out of feeling victimized, but since copping to feeling helpless is anathema to many otherwise powerful women, they quickly switch gears and become dedicated to attacking the one who has injured them.

Sometimes a sense of victimization can send a woman plummeting into a murky depression that, in the worst cases, produces suicidal despair. This victim prays for rescue from the partner whose love and capacity to see the error of his ways seems like all that stands between her and hopelessness. A true victim believes that only the one who has hurt her can protect her. She feels most real to herself in the dank, black cellar of the psyche, where she lays abandoned and bereft. Only a childhood of devastating pain or a seriously compromised neurochemistry that requires medication can thrust someone this far into victimhood for more than a few hours at a time. But if you do go there, even on the rarest of rare occasions, it's important to see how your agony serves you and understand why you insist upon locking yourself up in this cell. It isn't your lover who leaves you there and then walks away—it's you.

Your Obsession First Aid Kit: Set Yourself Free

Your Obsession First Aid Kit is packed with exercises that will help you overcome your romantic obsessions and:

- show you where your emotional sore spots are—the tender areas I call your "emotional Achilles' heel";
- help you quell your use of such reactive behaviors as the Sorry Six that keep your obsessions spinning;
- show you how to soothe your Achilles' heel and gain balance by replacing the Sorry Six with specific self-focused actions.

Now that you know which of the Sorry Six feel familiar, let's look at how the patterns might have originated.

A BLAST FROM YOUR PAST

In a moment I'm going to ask you to close your eyes and imagine yourself in the home where you grew up and to recall what you felt there. First, think about what you felt in response to the overall atmosphere in your household. The atmosphere could be considered the emotional climate. Some households have a hot, chaotic, unpredictable climate; others have a cool, restrained, rigid feel. Depending on the climate, you might have felt scared, uncertain, defensive, expectant, excited, gleeful, nervous, angry, etc. Second, I'd like you to think about how you felt about yourself as a youngster and teen. For instance, did you feel unwanted, superior, helpful, bad, special, loved, needed, unappreciated?

Go ahead and close your eyes, breathe deeply, and take yourself through the process I just described. When you've completed the exercise, write down all the feelings that came to mind.

Now, paying close attention to your awareness of all of these feelings, I'd like you to answer the following questions, preferably in your journal:

- What did you do to deal with your feelings about the emotional climate in your home?

For example, if you felt anxious, how did you try to soothe yourself? Did you spend all your time in a fantasy world, reading books—like I did? Did you play outside, or throw yourself into your homework? Did you forage in the fridge and stuff yourself? If you felt uncertain or emotionally unsafe (and kids growing up in financially troubled or maritally distressed households often do), how did you try bringing more certainty to your world? Did you weave stories about what might happen next? Did you eavesdrop on your parents to try to find out more than you were being told? Did you smoke a lot of weed so you wouldn't care so much about what happened?

- What did you do to handle the feelings you had about yourself?

For example, if you felt neglected, did you get into trouble to attract attention? Or did you try to be a good girl, mommy's little helper? If you felt bad about yourself, did you act out? Did you try to stave off bad feelings by concentrating on how mean others were and fantasizing revenge?

I want to assure you that there are no right or wrong answers here. There's no reason to be ashamed of any of your reactions. You were a kid, and you reacted to the emotional climate as best you could, like every child does.

Now, let's go back to the Sorry Six patterns I described in the previous section: pursuit, distance, conflict, triangulation, blaming, and victimization. In thinking about what you did to cope with your feelings as a child, see whether your behaviors fall into any of these categories. Chances are, they'll fit into a few of them, although you might find a bunch of behaviors clustered in one.

One of my therapy clients, Amanda, told me about feeling mostly fearful in her home because she never knew when her verbally abusive mother would begin a rampage. After one of her mother's poison-tongued onslaughts, she'd hide out in her room and write hate letters to her mom, which she'd later shred into confetti. In terms of the Sorry Six, she reacted primarily by blaming and feeling victimized. And you know what? As a child, blaming her mother was sanity-saving. It was a hell of a lot better than taking her mother's behavior personally and blaming herself. Indeed, she was a victim of her mother's unmanaged aggression, and unlike a lot of kids in that situation, she knew it.

You can probably guess where we're going next: That's right, we'll be comparing these patterns with those in your current relationships.

Back to the Present: Identifying the Emotional Climate of Your Relationship

Let's answer the same two questions with an eye toward your most recent love affair. If you like, you can run through this exercise with each of the important relationships in your romantic history. If you do, I promise that your diligence will pay off. Here's the process again:

1. Close your eyes, take a deep breath, and imagine yourself enveloped by your relationship as if it were a little universe with an atmosphere unto itself. What words best describe the emotional climate that surrounds you? Is it unstable, secure, chaotic, erratic, etc.?
2. What words best describe the way you feel about yourself in this relationship? Remember, this means feeling special, unloved, inferior, bitchy, superior, etc. Write all of these words in your journal.
3. Think about how you cope with this array of feelings. First, how do you contend with the emotional climate of the relationship; that is, how do you react to it, or what do you typically do to try to alter or control it?
4. Next, what do you do to cope with how you feel about yourself in this relationship?

5. Can you categorize any of the things you typically do as forms of pursuit, distancing, generating conflict, triangling, blaming, or victimizing yourself?

Take a moment to note your thoughts in your journal. By now you can probably see themes that have remained consistent across the years, as well as new areas of vulnerability and maneuvers you have devised for dealing with them.

Amanda, who wrote all those hate letters to her mom, discovered in doing this process that her hate letters to mom have grown up, too, and turned into lengthy, accusatory e-mail messages to her boyfriend. When she feels victimized by her lover, she writes a letter that she doesn't have to tear up, as she did all those years ago. She clicks the send button and feels more powerful for having had her say. Plus, she can express herself from a distance so that she isn't threatened by his immediate counterattack. She can shore up her defenses and read his response when she feels strong enough to handle it. Oh, the joys of technology.

BABE BOOSTER

Instead of driving yourself batty trying to figure out why your guy does the crazy things he does, stop and pay attention to the things you do!

Unfortunately, the elements that keep her in an obsessive loop have not changed. The anguished sense of being misunderstood, unfairly attacked, and, of course, her focus on *him* persist in the present. Whether her boyfriend is truly behaving the way her mother did is less important than the fact that Amanda expects him to act that way. She's on guard, so the emotional climate of her present-day world is surprisingly parallel to the one she knew as a child. Neither the hate letters to mom nor the achingly detailed letters to her boyfriend can provide real solace.

What might Amanda do instead? Most importantly, she could learn to create the solace that has so far escaped her. That might mean learning to meditate, involving herself in creative work that gives expression to her subtle gifts, or releasing some of her tension through real exercise rather than mental gymnastics. Amanda could begin to soothe and appreciate herself instead of hoping others will do that job for her, and then feel desolate when they fail. With her boyfriend, an unguarded expression of desire might be all the words she needs to turn the tide. Anything might happen if she says, "I really want to connect with you. I want to know you, and I want you to know me. Let's see how we can get better at that."

Coping with Your Emotional Achilles' Heel

We're all vulnerable to our partners in different ways. When our sore spots are kicked, we feel our anxiety go through the roof, and we react. We could consider our sorest of sore spots to be our emotional Achilles' heel. We're more likely to react strongly and immediately using the Sorry Six when an arrow lands in our Achilles' heel. In fact, it's fair to say that you never react unless you feel an "ouch."

The first step to acquiring self-focus is to catch yourself in mid-reaction…and STOP.

Just because you start an argument doesn't mean you have to keep fueling it. Just because you call your guy and hang up for the third time doesn't mean you have to pick up the phone the fourth time. Eventually, you'll learn to shift gears before you react at all—before you pull one of the Sorry Six out of your bag of tricks. But that's way down the road. *For now, when you hear yourself invoking one of the Sorry Six, just STOP.* Your Achilles' heel has taken a blow, your anxiety level is rising and there's only one thing to do: Breathe.

Yes, breathe. Deeply. In and out. Notice how anxiety feels in your body. Where is it lodged? Is your chest tight? Are your stomach muscles clenched? Is your jaw gripping? Is your "seat of anxiety" engaged (the muscle group that includes your sphincter, butt, abdominals, and lower back)?

You can clue your partner in by saying, "I didn't mean to react so strongly, can you give me a minute to get hold of myself?"

Keep breathing as you cleanse away tension and become present in your body, attentive to emotional and sensual experience. Let your breath enter through you nose, picturing its warmth loosening and stretching tight areas. Then, imagine you are blowing away stress as you slowly, steadily exhale through your mouth, pursed in the form of a loose "O."

By catching yourself mid-reaction and paying attention to your body, you can slow down enough to take the next step, which involves locating the emotion behind your reactivity. We'll do that by exploring three new questions. By answering them in your journal, you'll be well on your way to seeing your reactions in a new light.

Question One: What does your lover *say* and *do* that almost guarantees you'll launch into one of the Sorry Six? Write down at least five examples of times when he said or did something that kicked off one of the Six.

Let me show you what I mean with an example from my practice. When Donna finally drummed up the nerve to share a cherished sexual fantasy with Troy, he responded by scrunching up his nose and saying dismissively, "Oh well." If Donna had answered the previous question she would have said, "When I try to tell Troy something important, sometimes he dismisses me and I get really mad." Feeling dismissed is one of Donna's emotional Achilles' heels. In this instance, when Troy disregarded Donna's disclosure she reacted instantaneously by charging, "You're so damn conservative!"

Question Two: What do you actually *feel* at the moment when your lover says or does something that triggers one of the Sorry Six? Think back to the list you just made. What is the emotion that tends to precede your reaction to each? If you're tempted to say anger, look deeper. Anger is often a reaction to a feeling that's harder to contend with: hurt, guilt, envy, fear, shame, etc.

In Donna's case, even though she reacted angrily, she actually felt ashamed. When Troy recoiled, she assumed he found her fantasy revolting. In one split second, she saw the whole relationship unravel, certain that she'd revealed a dark, sticky, unlovable part of herself. But Donna didn't remain immersed in her shame—to do so would have been far too painful. She grew irritable instead, and when she pounced on Troy, he defended himself, saying: "I'm not conservative, you're the one! You think your fantasy is some big deal, but it's child's play!"

Now Donna felt foolish, and even more ashamed for revealing her lack of sophistication, but again, she couldn't stay with her feelings or reveal them. Instead, she retorted, "Well, if you're so cool, how come you hate it when I bring my vibrator to bed?"

Donna kept poking at Troy because she felt badly about herself. Yet, beneath her anger and blame crouched the raw shame she was avoiding—it was a feeling that had come and gone so quickly that she didn't have a chance to catch it by the tail before it was replaced with fury. And it was a much uglier sensation for Donna to accept than anger—it was her most tender Achilles' heel.

What could Donna have done instead of provoking conflict with Troy?

She could have slowed down long enough to see that her sorest spot had been poked. She could have viewed her very first use of one of the Sorry Six as a red flag. Right there, she could have said "Oops!" and stopped everything to look in the mirror at herself rather than through a magnifying glass at Troy. Then she would have had some interesting truths to explore. Donna might even have changed the entire tone of the discussion by saying, "I felt awful, Troy. First I was ashamed that you thought I was too kinky, then that you thought I wasn't kinky enough. I guess I really need to figure out how to feel good about my own sexuality so I don't need your approval one way or the other."

You might be thinking that speaking out would have meant taking quite a risk. Maybe Donna had every reason to feel unsafe sharing her shame with Troy, considering his tendency to be dismissive. But doesn't that line of thinking make this story all about Troy? And doesn't it imply that unless Troy makes the relationship comfy for Donna, she can't be authentic or bold?

A Babe does not buy into such ideas! Granted, if Troy couldn't listen respectfully, Donna would have to seriously examine that aspect of the relationship as well. But if she were to let his receptiveness determine whether she speaks from her heart or holds her tongue, then Donna would forfeit any chance at intimacy. After all, intimacy demands a certain transparency. That's why the word intimacy is often broken down and defined as "into-me-see." Sure, it's a stretch, but notice it's not broken down as "into-me-see-and-validate-me."

Now, let's get back to your questions. The one we're looking at is: How do you feel when your partner says or does something to trigger a flurry of reactivity? Be sure to jot the answer in your journal.

In light of Donna's story, do you see that nothing your partner actually says or does is the *basis* of your reactions? When you launch into one of the Sorry Six, you're actually reacting to the fact that your own emotional Achilles' heel has taken quite a hit—you're reacting to that pain, and the thoughts the hurt provokes.

Question Three: Under what circumstances do you try hardest to control your partner's behavior or reactions? Why? What is the feeling (shame, fear of loss, guilt, hurt, etc.) that you want to get out from under so badly that you'll use any psychological weapon at hand to control your partner?

The Obsessive Game

Obsessive love is a romantic game grounded in manipulating and controlling an external source of validation. If we can control our lovers so that we don't have to feel our own anguish—if we can stop him or her from behaving in ways that we associate with our nightmare sensations—then we win the game!

Being a Babe, being balanced and self-focused, means getting in on an entirely different game. We win when we can accept our own feelings, choose our own behaviors, and become responsible for the kind of love we invite into our life. The prize is not only a respectful, conscious relationship with ourselves, but is also, in all probability, a truly deep, rich, intimate relationship with another.

Four Steps Toward Balance

Having answered the last three questions, you're prepared to take the four steps that will lead you toward balance. The steps look simple on paper, but they're demanding. A Babe needs to practice like an Olympic gymnast competing for the gold.

1. Consider your use of any of the Sorry Six to be a red flag that your emotional Achilles' heel has taken a hit!
2. Say "Oops!" (or !#@!* will also do nicely) and *stop* reacting. Breathe deeply. Get your bearings. Remember, it's okay not to keep a reactive cycle going and going and going just because you started it. Pay attention to where your anxiety is lodged in your body. Use your breath to help relax the areas of tension. Inhale deeply through your nose, fill your chest, and then exhale very slowly though your mouth until you run out of air. Do this three to five times.

3. Once you've calmed down, think about the feelings associated with your anxiety (especially that one that flew by so fast! Grab it quick and hang onto it!).
4. Act in a new, self-focused way.

You've already done a lot of work in your journal to prepare you for tackling steps one through three. Next time you experience an episode of reactivity with your lover, try going back to your journal. You'll gain further insight by looking at the experience in light of the previous questions and noting your perceptions.

Now, let's look more closely at steps three and four.

Doing the Turtle Walk

A silly phrase came to me one day when I was thinking about how we put new behaviors into practice. The phrase is "like a turtle walks." I thought of the familiar parable of the tortoise and the hare, and how the tortoise won the race by being slow but steady. When we are jacked up on emotion in an obsessive romance, we tend to rush forward like the hare, quick to pursue, quick to flee, quick to fight—and just as quick to collapse. We need to become more tortoiselike, adopting a slower pace to allow ourselves time to think through our feelings, our words, our actions, and our capacity for self-care.

Replacing reflexive patterns with self-focused thoughts and behaviors requires practice and perseverance as you try out new approaches, discover what works for you and what doesn't, and make alternate selections. In essence, you slowly teach yourself a new vocabulary for responding to old provocations.

Since covering each of the Sorry Six individually could take up an entire book in itself, I'm going to take on the familiar style of pursuit and walk you through the process of gaining self-focus when all you want to do is chase after reassurance, validation, or the mere presence of your lover. Because the steps are exactly the same for all, you'll be able to apply what you learn to the gamut of the Sorry Six by adding your own creative twists.

GETTING BEYOND PURSUIT

In the sickening emptiness of one partner's distance, the other's pursuit begins. Repetitive phone calls, cards, letters, gifts, pleas for assurance, showing up at a lover's workplace or home, trying to be pleasing and compliant and then suddenly flying off the handle—these are the common efforts we make in pursuit. But even screaming, demanding, insisting, and accusing can be indirect forms of pursuit. Behind all of these is the same message: "Come to me...please!"

Naturally, in healthy relationships, pursuit can be a positive force. Mutual pursuit may mean striving toward a common goal or working to straighten out a problem together, sort of like an arts and crafts project where "you can be the paper and I'll be the scissors and our love will be the glue." The emotions behind mutual pursuit include hope, affection, appreciation, and generosity.

We usually know when a pursuit is genuinely loving and when it's obsessive. Obsessive pursuit is fueled by throat-tightening anxiety and desperation—it's all about take and take, not give and take. When you stop an obsessive pursuit cycle to check in with your authentic feelings, you see the little man behind the curtain wearing a T-shirt smeared with words such as fear, jealousy, outrage, hurt, and despair.

SOOTHING YOUR PURSUIT ANXIETY

Stop a moment and jot down a quick list of the types of actions you take when in pursuit. (If you never pursue, but instead always distance or start fights, go ahead and focus on what you do and follow all the next steps with your typical reactive style in mind.)

Imagine this: From now on, whenever you're tempted to pull pursuit ploys out of your knapsack, you'll *stop*, breathe deeply, and then locate the feeling behind the urge to pursue. You want to deal with *that* emotion rather than launch into your familiar reactive behavior. (Doesn't the very idea of being so aware feel calming—kind of like mental chocolate?) Since nine times out of ten you'll find one of the "nasty T-shirt" emotions I mentioned a moment ago, you'll need to do something that is both self-focused and continues to soothe your distress. Until now, you've been stifling that distress with pursuit ploys, but, Babe, those days are just about over.

Learning to identify emotions and soothe yourself is the height of balanced Babeness. I'm not suggesting that a Babe doesn't feel sadness, anxiety, desperation, or fear, only that being brave enough to accept those feelings and manage them wisely when they do arise is what separates the Babes from the boys!

Let's look at how the process might play out for Katy, who has been dating John for about three months and works herself up into pursuit frenzy when she hasn't heard from him in a few days. She gets most anxious after they've had bitter words or she thinks he might be out with another woman, since although they're steadies, they aren't yet exclusive. She usually stews for a few hours and then drives over to his house. Sometimes she just checks to see whether someone else's car is sitting in his driveway and sometimes she shows up all smiles at his door. It's a crapshoot to see whether John gets mad and sends her off into the night or invites her in to make up and make out.

Katy and John never solve the problems at the root of their obsessive relationship because they're too busy with instant replays of the same old game. To change the rules, Katy needs to stay out of John's neighborhood, literally and metaphorically. Katy can shift the focus from John to herself by taking the Four Steps Toward Balance that we've already talked about. She would begin by noticing that her Achilles' heel has taken a hit, and she'd stop reacting and take some deep breaths. Then, she'd move on to step three and step four.

STEP THREE: FOCUS ON FEELINGS
There are two aspects to this step: acknowledging your feelings and pointing to the faulty beliefs about yourself that underlie your feelings.

Katy might start by asking herself, "Which feelings are behind my urge to pursue right now?" As she attends to her emotional state, she might recognize the sense of abandonment and loss that overwhelms her when John is out of touch. She might hear a little voice inside her head murmuring frightful *what ifs*, such as "What if I lose him for good?" Recognizing that she is bound up in fear of rejection might remind her of all the other painful rejections throughout her life, and she might realize that she's actually reacting to the accumulated hurt of twenty-eight years, not just to two days of worry over lack of communication from John.

As Katy focuses on the beliefs associated with her feelings, she would begin to see that they represent catastrophic exaggerations of the current reality. Her critical inner voice might be creating a ruckus with thoughts such as: "I'm not good enough for John. He couldn't possibly want me because I'm not smart enough or pretty enough for someone like him. Surely he's out on the town, looking elsewhere."

Obsessive romances are fueled by a common set of belief patterns. These include: "I'm not lovable," "I'm not enough," "I can't survive alone," "I'm not safe," "People always fail me." All of these beliefs have one quality in common—they are false!

Even if there is a kernel of truth to any of these words (for example, maybe some people *have* failed you in the past), the extent of truth is always disproportionate to the enormous volume of the lie. When we make emotional choices based on a lie of such magnitude, how worthy can those choices be?

STEP FOUR: ACT IN A NEW, SELF-FOCUSED WAY

This step has two components: replacing negative beliefs with positive ones and sensory self-soothing.

You may not be able to do both at any given time. Whether you're alone or engaged in a dialogue with your partner will make a difference, too. You get to decide which approach is wisest. However, when in doubt, start with self-soothing. Sensory soothing will buy you time, keep you from reacting prematurely, and improve the emotional climate of your personal universe.

Let's take the components of step four one by one.

Replace Negative Beliefs with Positive Beliefs

Feeling as badly about herself as she does, Katy might feel almost compelled to rush out and see John to soothe her fears. Instead, if she is to make any lasting gains, Katy needs to hang on to herself, stay put, and focus on countering the negative beliefs that are running roughshod through her mind. She needs to seek the competent, desirable part of herself and remind herself why she deserves love, appreciation, and most of all, compassion for herself and from herself. This is reparative work for Katy, and critical to ending the obsessive cycle.

Katy might have to remind herself that even though she seems to fall apart at the slightest provocation in relation to John, she is also strong and competent in her work, and she is a loyal, caring friend. She might need to say to herself, "I am worthy of love and attention. I am bright and kind and a pleasure to be with."

Replacing negative beliefs with positive ones isn't done in a flash—it's an ongoing effort. Usually negative beliefs are already entrenched, and a genuine shift in belief patterns takes time. All of the work can't be done as you are feeling an urge to react with one of the Sorry Six. In Katy's case, it might be enough to keep from grabbing the car keys and running out the door. She might not be able to settle down quickly enough to focus on anything but the urge to pursue. Sometimes the effort to change beliefs has to be made later, when you're past the danger of acting out and can take time to sort through and think about your cycles.

If the heat of the moment is too great, you'll find a safe haven in resuming breathing—deep, healing breaths—so that the oscillating waves of tension can stabilize and flow from your body. Turning to sensory self-soothing now will keep you grounded in your body and detached from the familiar loop of obsessive rumination and reactive behaviors.

Discover the Bliss of Sensory Self-Soothing

The work that you do to connect with your feelings and beliefs is one layer of the process of breaking free of obsession. Another layer involves supporting that process with loving, calming behaviors that nurture your spirit and caress your soul. These take you beyond concentration on the relationship altogether. I call this sensory self-soothing—the adult equivalent of being rocked and sung a lullaby as an infant. When you are tempted to pursue—or engage in any of the other Sorry Six—and you have a tough time focusing on feelings and beliefs, sensory self-soothing is your first line of defense. Sometimes it's best to remain entirely outside your own head where repetitive, negative thoughts and troubling impulses reside.

The more you rely on sensory self-soothing for anxiety reduction, the less you'll need to use one of the Sorry Six as a fail-safe mode of coping with disturbing emotions. Sensory self-soothing should be done mindfully; that is, with full attention given to each act. If you're petting your dog, feel the soft texture of his coat, the rise and fall of his chest as he inhales and exhales. If you're baking bread, immerse yourself in each detail—the texture of the flour, the aroma of melted butter. You want to train yourself to move beyond the habit of doing one thing with your body while your mind remains hopelessly fixated on the object of your obsession. How many times have you said to yourself, "How did I get here?" because you were driving the car or puttering around the house on autopilot while your mind was absorbed in the alternate universe of relationship strife. Such is the opposite of mindfulness.

Here are a dozen suggestions for sensory self-soothing. The options are limitless, though. See if you can add a few more ideas that are uniquely yours:

- Light a candle and watch the flame.
- Go out in the middle of the night and watch the stars.
- Listen to beautiful or soothing music, or to invigorating and exciting music.
- Give attention to the sounds of nature (waves, birds, rainfall, leaves rustling).
- Bake cookies, cake, or bread.
- Walk in a wooded area and breathe in the fresh smells of nature.
- Treat yourself to a dessert.
- Pet your dog or cat.
- Rent a favorite movie.
- Go for a massage.
- Soak your feet.
- Put creamy lotion on your whole body.
- Hug someone.

As you learn to become mindful in soothing anxiety and drawing back from the Sorry Six, your romantic obsessions will lose steam. At that point, to drive your relationship toward intimacy and excellence, you'll need to give it serious attention and, with your partner, develop enhanced skills for connection. That work—the work of two—is beyond the scope of this book. However, in the resource section I will direct you to the best material I know to assist in your growth as a couple.

But here's the rub: When you place your emphasis on becoming balanced—not on getting a certain response from your partner that reintroduces a state of agitated fusion—you may wind up deeply disappointed in your partner's ability to function as an equal in the relationship. You may be forced to confront the very truth about the relationship that you had been dreading.

Sometimes obsessive behaviors keep a dead relationship alive by inciting drama. When you stop the drama and detach from the action, you may discover that there is nothing substantial there, or you may find that your partner can't meet you at your level. Some relationships are not meant to be, and the more balanced and authentic you become, the more willing you are to accept that fact. Neither all the obsessive acting out, nor all the healthy balanced behavior in the world, will make a prince out of a frog or create a match between two people who are simply unmatchable. This is perhaps the hardest lesson to learn and may cause pain for which there is no real cure except time—and the belief that something better awaits you. However, as you stay busy working on yourself, you also make yourself ready for the high-quality relationship you deserve.

CHAPTER 4

Release the Shame, Unleash the Slut

Get dirty without feeling guilty

REMEMBER DONNA in the last chapter, who felt such shame when her husband dismissed her sexual fantasy? It breaks my heart to think of all the Donnas in this world who are unable to celebrate the wonder of their erotic imaginations. Yet I am comforted by the knowledge that each "Donna" has everything she needs within herself to break free of her tethers and become a vibrantly powerful Babe.

Becoming a Babe begins with being willing to dig down into yourself, find your hidden cache of shame, and empty it—one repressive thought, one painful memory at a time. Being a Babe may mean becoming radically bold—acting as if you have no shame at all, knowing that if you believe you are entitled to live as a free spirit, your authentic self and your actions will win out over any forces that might otherwise hold you back.

EXERCISE Rewriting Your Sexual Script

In our families, we are all exposed to an early sexual narrative. Sometimes that exposure is overt, sometimes covert. In Julie's family, sex was a hush-hush matter, as even lightly risqué jokes were frowned upon. Yet, from the time she was eight until she was thirteen, her father made a practice of drinking too much and then slipping into her bed late at night to fondle her and, as time wore on, force her to fondle him. The "truth" about sex that Julie learned at her father's hand? Sex is a furtive and forbidden act.

In Janis's family, sexuality was displayed freely. "Dirty" jokes were dinner table conversation. By the age of twelve, she was allowed to watch her parents' adult videos along with them. Her mother dressed in tight, low-cut clothing and her father's hands roamed his wife's body as he pleased. Janis's lesson? Sex is hot, dirty, and fun; anything goes, anytime, anywhere. A woman should be available at all times for her man's pleasure.

Think about the way sex was regarded in your family. What is the script that weaved its way through your experience? In a sentence or two, what is the "truth" about sex you learned in your childhood home? If you would like to revise that lesson, write down the new truth with which you would like to replace the old. What do *you* need to do differently in order to bring your new truth to life?

The Shame About Shame

Contemporary Western culture has few rituals for initiating girls into womanhood. While young women in many tribal societies are ceremonially ushered into adulthood, the closest we come on a broad scale is to herd wide-eyed teens into junior high school gymnasiums where they are shown moralistic or medical films about their changing bodies. This tainted introduction to femininity lacks even passing reference to the beauty and sacredness of their blossoming sexuality.

BABE BOOSTER

It takes a five to one ratio of positive to negative interactions to make a relationship work. Your sexual-self demands the same.

We grow up exposed to negative concepts about our sex and our bodies that leave an indelible mark. The shame that is inculcated early remains inside, sabotaging our grown-up choices until we excise that shame core by our own hand.

If sex were paired only with shame, we'd be sure to succumb to the abundance of sex-negative messages, but strangely enough, our saving grace is found in being dealt confusing mixed messages. Sex may be bad, dangerous, or sinful, but it's also thrilling, tantalizing, ultra-cool, and advertised everywhere. On the one hand, young women are convinced that to be wanted they must look like sirens in belly-button bearing fashion, all plump juicy mouth and skinny busty body—on the other hand, born-again virgins believe that sexual anorexia is a healthy extreme.

Shaky as they are, we do have options!

Nevertheless, shame's hushed presence distorts our relationship with ourselves and thwarts the potential for deep intimacy with others. Shame makes us hesitant to communicate sexual or emotional needs, lest we provoke a partner's disdain. Shame may lead us to act unsafely, choosing partners who are emotionally vacant, hurtful, or controlling, in an effort to deny our confusion about our desires. Shame may force us to compensate for sexual abandon, for guilty pleasures, by overcontrolling other urges. We may seek the hollowness of anorexia, the bloat of bulimia, compulsive exercise, or any self-restraint taken to dangerous extremes in an attempt to cancel out our wantonness. Shame may even demand we erect a wall of denial around our sexual activity and so fail to protect ourselves from disease or pregnancy. In these ways, we sabotage our health and our self-esteem—but it's shame that is the monster, not our sexuality, not our excitement-seeking.

OH, TO BE A SLUT

In one of my most recent columns for *Men's Fitness* magazine, I replied to a letter from a newly married man whose bride had confessed that she had lied about her sexual näiveté before their marriage. He was in a quandary over how to react to both pieces of the new equation—her sexual experience, and her lie. I understood his consternation but couldn't help reacting to the idea that fear had driven her to deny her rich history in the first place. Had he set her up by belittling women of experience? If so, why hadn't she told him to take a hike instead of lying and tying the knot? But, of course, her decision to hide the truth and validity of her own experience and hang on for dear life to her marital prospect didn't come out of the blue—or even out of her relationship with this particular man. Undoubtedly, it was the fruit of a shame-seed that had been planted some twenty years earlier when she was first initiated into the mysteries of womanhood; a seed that burst open when she hit her sexual stride and discovered that even at the turn of the twenty-first century, nice girls don't.

Along the same lines, I was paging through a *Glamour* magazine in my dentist's office and came upon the monthly "Let's Talk About Sex" feature in which a group of women—including a few celebrity types—sit around dishing various hot topics. In this case, it was the matter of the one-night stand: should we or shouldn't we? The consensus among the gals was that one-nighters have their place in a woman's need-fulfilling repertoire. That said, one woman piped up, "Then why do we still feel such shame about it?" Good question! No doubt because every one of those advocates had that shame drummed into her since she was old enough to grasp the notion that a one-night stand is a man's prerogative and a woman's game of chance; if Mr. Booty doesn't call again, she is an instant slut—just add hot water and stir. Only if the phone rings is she spared.

Babe Is the Only Label That Applies

A Babe does not for a minute allow herself to be held hostage to latter-day notions about what makes her a good girl, a bad girl, a saint, or a slut. If forced to choose one of those labels, a Babe would naturally pick slut, and then in a nanosecond reframe it, maybe give it an acronym of its own—*Sexy, Loving, Uninhibited, Truthful.* Actually, a Babe finds that all such labels, including the hip use of "bad girl" so popular in books and glib lifestyle manuals these days, divides women from one another when we most need each other's support. Besides, a Babe is not a girl, "bad" or otherwise. She's a woman: a bodacious and sometimes quite brazen W-O-M-A-N.

The Paradox of Desire

In the eighties, when the movement toward sexual equality was gathering so much steam, I remember hoping that by the turn of the century we'd be past the point of needing analysis of why women can't soar freely in their sexual power. To my dismay, we're well past that point in time but not in progress, for women's relationship to desire itself still remains skewed. Blatant sexual imagery drenches the airwaves, saturates the pages of magazines, and drips from pop-up windows in every corner of cyberspace. Despite all this wet 'n' wild action, the cultural conditions that simultaneously idolize the female sexual body and thwart active female desire are almost as firmly in place as they were before the sexual revolution of the sixties. Women, the exalted objects of male lust, are still raised to deny their own desire. How paradoxical that we are born to be symbols of the very urge that we are expected to abstain from exploiting for our own joy!

In *Sex and Single Girls* (one of the best books available on being an erotically alive woman in today's world), Tara Hardy contributes an essay called *Femme Dyke Slut* in which she grapples with the contradiction of being lesbian and outrageously feminine when the zeitgeist demanded allegiance to butchness or androgyny, the antithesis of all that was traditionally female. Hers was the corollary to the straight woman's effort to be a babe in the traditional, cutesy sense—pleasing to the male eye rather than pleasing to herself. Instead of seeing ourselves as the living force from which desire emanates, when we gaze into a mirror, we see the source of male fulfillment staring back.

This paradox reinforces our attraction to obsessive relationships. As I mentioned in Chapter 2, when you feel yourself merging, melting into the delirium of fused love, you can't separate your own desire from your lover's. You can, however, manage a guiltless flood of desire as your lover's hunger meets yours. Does it matter who is the source of desire, so long as you can ride the crest of it? Is it any wonder that you resist letting go of obsession? So long as you feel his craving as your own, your sexuality appears to thrive unhampered, and if this is all you know of desire—as it is for so many women—why trust that beneath this united rapture

BABE BOOSTER

Always remember this: Lovemaking is sorcery—you invoke power with the mere brush of a kiss.

there awaits a separate, equally profound core of desire all your own? In obsession, the basic (and otherwise obvious) fact that you can't feel your own needs through someone else's desire is obscured, and you remain one degree of separation away from touching the deeper fount of eroticism that is yours alone.

How do you locate this illusive wellspring of desire? Maybe you stumble upon a book like this one that takes you by the hand and shows you step by step, as I will do shortly, how to cull this power from within. Or maybe you've inadvertently come upon your desire. If you have, how does it feel? Alive and pulsating, like another heartbeat? Confusing, scary, threatening?

Maybe all of those things.

Sometimes our sexual needs and our capacity for pleasure frighten us. If we flaunt our sexuality, we fear those horrid labels. The more enmeshed we are with our families and our peers, the harder it is to relinquish culturally prescribed expectations about sex and intimacy. Being a self-focused Babe means choosing to be a blank slate and rediscovering our sexuality. A Babe doesn't give a hoot about prohibitions—she develops her own principles from the ground up and makes sexual choices that are consistent with her desires, seeking neither to comply with nor rebel against social or relational pressures. "This is who I am," she says simply, via her actions.

Gender Equality

Think about the differences between the way men and women view sexual power and entitlement. For example:

- Men don't loathe their bodies; women do.
- Men masturbate frequently; women don't.
- Men orgasm nearly every time they make love; women don't.
- Men don't need to learn how to have orgasms; women do.
- Men freely seek out, look at, and enjoy sexual imagery; women don't.
- Men don't fault themselves when a sexual encounter fails to become a dating relationship; women do.
- Men accept their bodies even if their weight exceeds the ideal; women don't.
- Men are comfortable displaying, touching, and assigning cute nicknames to their genitals; women aren't.

Make a point of initiating a discussion about this topic next time you are out with a group of women friends. You'll have a lively conversation and the other women will appreciate the opportunity to vent. We often don't realize how much we long for a place to share our thoughts about sexuality with other women until we create that space.

Commandeering Babe Power

For those women who are eager to grow as sexual beings, there has been some guiding progress over the past twenty or so years. Sex activists and feminist firebrands have helped to unclasp the average woman's chastity belt so that gals coming of age today have more latitude than did women who grew up in the fifties or sixties. But even twenty- to thirty-year-olds lack an inherited ease with which to express sexual curiosities and impulses. Condemnation and the double standard live on.

A Babe can count the ways these forces poke their nose into her bedroom and mess with the minds of the men she might want to love someday. A Babe immersed in the frantic single's scene is aware that some of the men she dates harbor archaic attitudes about chicks who are quick to be sexual, believing, circa 1950, that a woman who jumps into bed on the second or third date isn't the kind of girl one marries. (While their own studly behavior is above reproach.) Just the other day on a popular television talk show, the psychologist-host let a man excuse his reluctance to have leisurely, hot sex with his hapless, horny wife by running the tired old Madonna/whore syndrome past him. The sweet guy didn't want the saintly woman he married, the pure mother figure, to be "dirtied!" Yes, he said the word *dirty*!

> **BABE BOOSTER**
> *The next time you see someone you find attractive, look at him all over. Linger where you like, meet his gaze, hold his gaze, longer.... Make him look away first.*

Did the male host get in this guy's face and insist he (and millions of viewers, by the way) start to get real about the social conditions responsible for such shamefully skewed ideas about women, love, and sex? Uh uh. Oh, the doc did a nice job of addressing the nuances of their private relationship stuff, but he didn't clean up the "dirt," and I wondered whether that might not be because down deep, in his own southern gentleman psyche, the host's gray matter was flooded with the same toxic waste.

A Babe recognizes these outmoded, patronizing (and patriarchal) attitudes, but instead of kowtowing to them through her acquiescence, she acts from her own integrity, making love with whomever she chooses, whenever *she* is ready. "Any man who judges me for sharing myself with him," says one self-confident Babe, "is surely not a man I want to spend my life with! But, I still might want to sleep with him once or twice," she winks. A Babe knows that no one can make her feel ashamed, no one's censure can humiliate her—can even touch her—unless she believes she deserves condemnation.

As a Babe leaves obsessive romances behind, as her self-focus expands, that focus includes her scalding-hot sexual self. She attends to her emotional inner world, and yes, she focuses on her pussy, too! A Babe feels entitled to possess her eroticism and make authentic sexual choices with fearless joy. Instead of living up to the standards set by others, she lives up to standards derived from within.

If you want Babe power, here is what you will need to do:

• Be willing to point your finger at the insidious beliefs that suppress your sexual vitality;

• Peel away limiting thoughts about yourself;

• Make sexual choices with *your own passionate self-interest at heart*.

This means doing the one thing that is oh-so-basic, yet ever-so-tough —having sex strictly for your own pleasure or out of your own curiosity. Not just to bond, not to comply, not because you don't know how to say no, not because it's expected, not to be popular, not for your lover, but only because you want it.

As Babes, we can taste passion as if it were two dozen pints of Ben and Jerry's and choose our own favorite flavors. By supporting each other's sexual choices, no matter how ordinary or unique, we are supporting our female right to power. In this way, Babes are revolutionary forces to be reckoned with.

EXERCISE Making an "Unleash the Power" Collage

For this exercise, you'll need a few sheets of writing paper, one large sheet of construction paper, scissors, glue, and a pile of old magazines.

Begin by recalling all the restrictive, negative messages and beliefs you've absorbed over the years that have inhibited your sense of sexual self-esteem and erotic freedom. These may have come from your peers, your church, your family, the media, or your own experience of relationships. Take a clean sheet of writing paper and draw a line down the middle. On the left side of the line, write down all of your inhibiting beliefs. For instance:

• A good girl doesn't have sex until she falls in love.

• Men don't respect women who sleep around.

• Sex isn't all it's cracked up to be.

• Women want love; men want sex.

• You can't be smart and sexy; you have to be one or the other.

• Sex is a sacred act; casual sex is demeaning.

• To keep a man you have to give him what he wants in bed.

• Having sex during your period is gross.

By dumping this mass of sex-negative messages from your mind onto paper, you are taking the first step toward ridding yourself of their clutter and diluting their power to affect you.

When you've finished your list, on the other side of the center line, directly across from each old belief, compose a new, sex-positive statement that forcefully contradicts the negative one. You don't have to wholly subscribe to the new belief yet—you only need to conceive of it.

For example, next to "Sex isn't all it's cracked up to be" you might write, "As I teach myself about my body and learn the secrets of my pleasure, lovemaking becomes an ever-more thrilling adventure."

In contrast to "Only beautiful women are desirable" you might write, "I am gorgeous in the throes of passion, and when I cry out in delight at my lover's touch, he finds me irresistible."

Neatly copy all of the new, self-affirming statements onto a fresh, unlined sheet of paper.

Now you're ready to create your collage. Gather up the magazines and flip through the pages, seeking images you find erotically or sensually provocative. Clip them out and combine your handwritten statements and the photographs you've chosen on the large sheet of construction paper in any pattern that pleases you.

Take your time with this project, and with each phrase or photo that you glue onto the collage, assure yourself that you are exchanging a shameful or limiting vision for one that is bursting with possibility.

When you're done, place your creation in a position of honor in your home. You will be reminded daily of the erotic power and promise that is newly at the center of your world.

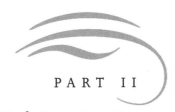

PART II

Cultivating Ecstasy:
Having the Sex Life You Deserve

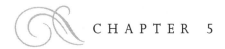

CHAPTER 5

Our Erotic Seventh Sense

Harness your erotic energy and take it for a ride

S
OME YEARS BACK, I took a driving trip along the rugged northeast coast. I was hoping to find the perfect place to cocoon for a while and write.

Just outside of Blue Hills, Maine, I stumbled upon a carriage house attached to a charming resort called the Eggemoggin Reach Inn. I remember catching my breath as I first entered the cottage—it was idyllic. The interior was crafted in rich, warm cherry wood, and its cathedral ceilings and expansive windows gave it a feeling of vast space. Nestled in the pine forest, it overlooked a bay with a view of the tiny Pumpkin Island lighthouse blinking in the distance. I had found my dream home—no, it was better than I could have dreamed!

I had been there for about a week, already dreading leaving, when very late one night a storm rose up, seemingly out of nowhere. The wind howled, heavy raindrops pelted the roof. Soon the howling became a low throaty roar, as though a fantastical beast were circling my fairy-tale cottage.

I had been clicking away at the computer, wearing only a light filmy robe—now I stood up and headed for the French doors that led to the balcony. As I urged them open, the wind slammed them backward with such might that I let out a little yelp; the doors crashed against the adjacent walls, the glass panes rattled in their grids. I stepped onto the balcony, as my hair whipped around my face and my robe flew open, baring my flesh. All of the elements raged and I stood in awe of the ferocious beauty. Then, just as quickly as the storm had risen, it waned. In the sudden quiet I gazed across the moonlit water, the butterfly wings of my robe floating behind me, and a soft breeze began caressing my body like the fingertips of a lover. I sighed, and leaning into the currents of air, I allowed my breasts and shoulders to be stroked. My nipples grew hard, yearning. I closed my eyes, slowed my breathing, arched my back and gave in to this gentle lover. I let the wind and the raindrops and the scent of pine and sea take me. I was all sensation— no thought, really—but so thoroughly aroused that I shuddered. And then, without warning—just like that—the moment passed, the wind stilled entirely, and my lover departed. The thrall was broken, but the mood lingered like a kiss.

BABE BOOSTER

Make a concerted effort to seek out your eroticism and bring it home. Revel in the crackling sensations it creates in your life.

That night in Maine stands out as one of the most erotic moments in my memory, yet I had no sex, no sexual fantasy, no sexual partner.

So…what is this thing we call "the erotic?" Are we speaking of a mysterious force? An unruly impulse? A primal urge?

I see eroticism as all of these and more. Eroticism is so thoroughly a sieve through which life experience is poured that to call it a force or an impulse is not quite immense or encompassing enough. Eros is as integral to our means of perceiving as touch, as sight, as hearing, as taste, as scent, and at the same time, our eroticism hinges on all of these.

A Multiplicity of Senses

Do we really have a sixth sense? Most of us have experienced moments of intuitive brilliance or psychic awareness that defy analysis yet can't be explained away. If it's true that we have a sixth sense that reaches into the paranormal realm, isn't it possible that we have a seventh sense? Even an eighth or a ninth?

The erotic encompasses a knowing so acute that it comes closest to being a sense: a particular, unified way of ripping our world into titillating, often astonishing tidbits and reassembling them into patterns of meaningful experience.

Our erotic sense is desire's faithful and necessary companion. To feel the flow of desire, we need only to tune into the erotic stimulants swirling around us. They are ever present if we remain still long enough to be ravished by them. Unlike the visual or auditory sense, our erotic sense isn't primarily tied to one organ system—it incorporates many. The erotic lives in the realm between sensuality and sexuality, between imagination and action, between being and thinking. The erotic prevails upon our five key senses, endlessly taunting them; it is both of our bodies and of our psyches, of our present and of our past. To attempt to control our eroticism is to try to control the perceptual foundation of being alive. To fear our eroticism is tantamount to fearing touch or vision or taste.

A Babe gives her erotic sense a place of honor at the center of her world.

One of the advantages of viewing eroticism as a sense rather than as a force is that our senses are value-neutral. We don't judge the fact that we have a visual sense or an auditory sense or a sense of taste. We do, however, observe certain cautions with respect to how we use our senses. We don't play with fire, we don't eat things that have been in the trash, we don't look into the sun during an eclipse. If we embrace the erotic as part of our filigree of senses, one of the gifts of being human, we can relinquish some of the inbred guilt and shame over our erotic feelings—no matter what stimulates them. We can also give greater voice to our personal choices by asking: Does this behavior enrich me? Is it harmful? The danger of blocking out a sense would be obvious if we were speaking of one of the basic five. The danger of erotic denial is no different. We dare not barricade this doorway.

A Celebration of Sensation

The erotic is associated with the sexual, yet erotic experience can be a source of acute pleasure quite apart from the overtly sexual, and sexual behavior can be devoid of eroticism altogether. If you've even once had "mercy sex" to appease a horny partner when sex was the last thing on your mind, you understand this.

As my night in Maine illustrates, some of our most erotically vivid moments may be about the smallest detail of wind or rain, urgent music, soul-stirring art, or decadent Epicurean feasts. The banquet scene in the classic movie *Tom Jones* is flagrantly erotic, but there is no sex in it at all.

In Maine, it occurred to me that the erotic connection to nature is a primal one for women, producing a rawness of desire, a feeling of being one with the elements that peels away our civilized veneer and strips us down to a core of creaturely hungers. I was so convinced that this was a feminine phenomenon that I was unprepared for my boyfriend's reaction when I told him the story.

"I understand," he said. "I masturbated to a flower once."

I laughed, certain he was teasing me, but he was sincere. He told me of hiking in the mountains and coming across a vast field of wildflowers. The beauty of one bright flower in particular stood out. As he looked into the center where her petals joined, he became aroused, and right there, beneath the eyes of the sky, holding the gaze of his flower girl, he stroked himself until he came.

EXERCISE Tune into Your Seventh Sense

Think for a moment about your own erotic sense. How finely tuned is it? In your journal, write down as many erotic—but not overtly sexual—episodes as you can recall, and describe how you felt about them. Did they excite you, frighten you, leave you feeling out of control? Did they make you crave more? Make a commitment to yourself to choose one person with whom you can have a conversation about eroticism and share your experiences. Giving them voice is part of revealing yourself authentically, developing pride in your erotic sense, and supporting other women in doing the same.

I've been speaking of nonsexual erotic experiences. Few stand out in my mind with the detail of the storm in Maine. However, when I shift focus and search my memory for times when high eroticism coexisted with overt sexual energy—but no sexual *acts*—the stories practically trip over themselves vying to be told.

Straight off the top, I recall the night that my lover (yes, the flower man) and I stood opposite one another in my kitchen leaning against the two flanks of my U-shaped counter, and for nearly an hour, without ever touching, brought a sexual fantasy to life through words alone. He spoke of what he wanted to do with me, to me; I spoke of how I'd respond and what I'd do in return. By the time we stopped, I was so weak with arousal that my knees had begun to buckle. Did we rush headlong for the bedroom? No, we were due to meet friends for dinner, so we stepped out into the real world. Throughout the night we had only to glance at one another and, sure enough, kaleidoscopic fragments of our fantasy began twirling in our minds.

Sharpening Your Erotic Sense

Your erotic sense, like any other sense, can be sharpened through attention and attunement. I'm not inherently more sexual or more responsive than other women, and I'm certainly no less inhibited. But just as some women have an ear for music and others have a delicate palate, able to distinguish a chardonnay with vanilla and tropical notes from one with citrus undertones, I can shift into an erotic mode with a certain alacrity only because I have chosen to make that sense significant.

Any woman can celebrate the bounty of erotic pleasures in her life— if she wants to.

A Babe wants to.

Let's enjoy a little practice session right now.

EXERCISE Your Erotic Confession

Settle into a comfortable chair, or lie down and close your eyes. Make sure you won't be interrupted for a while. Let your mind wander over the images, the words, the sounds that you find most erotic in literature, media, music, and life. What stirs you? What pushes your buttons like nothing else?

Another way of looking at the question is to think back upon the most erotic moments in your experience and consider the conditions that made them especially passionate or sensual. Recall the atmosphere, the emotional tone, the words spoken, the scents, the way you felt about yourself and your lover, the tension or suspense, the sexual acts themselves, your aggressiveness or passivity, the aftermath.

Perhaps your erotic thoughts when you masturbate are more thrilling than anything you've known with a partner. Perhaps your erotic feelings are strongest when you imagine scenes that couldn't possibly occur in real life—like my friend who has a recurring dream of being ravished by the *Star Trek* character Worf. Take your time luxuriating in erotic thoughts and imagery. The outcome of this exercise is far less important than the process. Don't be afraid to touch yourself intimately during the exercise, as being aroused will help set the mood. When you're ready, open your eyes, take out your journal and begin to write your erotic "confession." Answer these questions:

What is the truth about you as an erotic creature? What surprises you, delights you, shocks you, frightens you about yourself? What is your secret to unleashing a rush of erotic feeling?

You can write a complete narrative, a poem, a series of phrases, words in a string—whatever feels right to you.

Writing your confession might feel strange at first, so, again, relax and luxuriate. Most of us aren't accustomed to making these revelations at all, much less in writing. We usually confess only to intimates and, even then, often as mere tossaways over a drink or two, accompanied by shy glances and nervous laughter. Rarely do we treat the cushy details of our erotic life like an overstuffed chair and then invite others to sink down into it. Most of the time we forbid ourselves the joy of lingering there, too, which is why doing this exercise is essential. It's all about curling up in your erotic world and giving substance to experiences you ordinarily let pass you by.

Playing Devil's Advocate

Why do I insist that a Babe place the erotic at the center of her world? If you wanted to play devil's advocate, wouldn't you ask why ordinary, satisfying sex when the planets are properly aligned isn't good enough? Besides, aren't there more important matters to consider as we look around this globe and see war, terror, poverty, hunger, and all manner of pain? Isn't this matter of erotic attention a bit self-indulgent?

Sure, you could make the case that concentrating on the erotic—on sex itself when not for purposes of procreation—is an indulgence reserved for a privileged few, and you'd receive no argument from me. Those of us who live in countries where resources are plentiful and support for human rights includes respect for sexual health and freedom are not only privileged indeed, but we are also in a position to actively make a difference in other corners of the world. But that doesn't mean we should reject the blessings we have.

I believe that a woman's eroticism flows like a living stream of creative, generative power within her. For this reason, rejoicing in the erotic is about more than momentary thrills or casual pleasures—it's about accessing your reservoir of sexual-spiritual energy.

To be engaged with the world fully, to draw upon your creative gifts, you need to touch the soul of your sex. Your erotic energy connects your values and desires to your actions—including your actions for justice in the world. You can't afford to make space for sexual guilt, for intimidation, for fear of your own ecstasy. The world needs your ecstasy far too much.

Ecstasy empowers you. Its opposite depletes you. When you have sex on borrowed desire, sex that is unwanted or demeaning, you devitalize yourself. And when you sap your energies, you are left with less to offer your loved ones, your community, your society.

A Babe has no room and no time in her life to relinquish or deplete her power. Let's look more closely at the nature of eroticism in our lives. How are we rewarded for developing this mysterious, yet awesomely powerful, seventh sense?

The Erotic Invites Self-Discovery

When we expose the erotic, we raise the shade on our inner life. Each of us has an erotic story to tell, a narrative that encompasses all that we fear, deny, yearn for, hate, and love. You wrote part of your narrative a moment ago, when you made your erotic confession.

There is nothing meaningless about our erotic narratives. They speak of our essential self more than the physicality of sex. When we reveal a desire, we expose a dream, filled with symbolism and substance, that tells us everything we need to know about who we are. The erotic is often lodged so deep in shadow that once we brave erotic revelations, there are no crimes left to hide from ourselves. First we face the truth, then we share our truth with others. As we timidly expose our erotic secrets, we become free. Authenticity flowers.

Owning and sharing our eroticism is the ultimate antidote to shame—for shame cannot survive exposure. It bursts into flame in the sunlight. Even shame too terrible to contemplate cannot suffer the light. One of the most important roles I play as a therapist is that of sister-confessor. When Angela speaks of the awe and excitement she felt at ten when her father forced his throbbing penis into her mouth, when Maria whispers of wanting to rape her lover, when Donella divulges the thrill she felt when her husband slapped her just that once, shame spills forth. As I listen and contain the secret, yet never blanch, Donella can hear herself, accept herself, and as the light of her acceptance mingles with the light of my witnessing, shame burns to cinders.

This is how shame dies. Not with tricks of logic, not by being rubbed between our thoughts until it's worn thin and flimsy, but by being driven out into air and sunlight. This is the power of support groups and women's groups and friendships. As even unspeakable secrets emerge, the self that felt soiled comes clean.

EXERCISE Share an Erotic Secret

Choose one person you trust and tell him or her something of emotional resonance that you've never shared before. You needn't reveal your most closely held secret, just one memory you've never spoken of before. For instance:

Coreen: "When I was eleven or twelve, I'd go into my father's closet and take his neckties to wear when no one was home. I played with myself while I wore them."

Donna: "Once, when I was nine, I got in bed with my best friend and showed her how to 'make herself tingle' down there, because she said she didn't know how."

Shannon: "This neighbor boy made me go down in his basement and show him my tits. I never tattled because I liked the game. Then one day I refused to take off my blouse until he pulled down his pants. He did it. That's when I knew I had power, too."

The Erotic Is a Wellspring of Creativity

The word erotic derives from the Greek word *eros* and refers to the god who personifies love, creative power, and harmony. This means that even in classical terms the erotic is about feeling deeply with all of our being—it's about living from our creative center and acting from the source of life itself.

Earlier I spoke of the erotic stream that flows within us as the source of creativity. We see evidence of this stream all around us: women creating art, writing music, rearing children, creating culture. Sometimes we see evidence in the unexpected encounter. I saw it in Nadja Solerna-Sonnenberg, and I'd like to tell you about her.

Nadja is a concert violinist of brilliance and acclaim. However, it isn't just her music that captivates me—it's her face. Should I ever come to doubt that the erotic sense is a fount of creative expression, I have only to watch Nadja at her instrument to be reassured.

When Nadja plays the violin, she *is* sex. She is eroticism. Nadja has been criticized by traditional reviewers for showing too much ferocious expressiveness. In the documentary, *Speaking in Strings*, Nadja refers to love as the smallest part of her life, though on her Web site recently, she mentioned being "completely consumed" romantically. Whatever is or is not happening in her heart offstage, with her chin pressed hard against the edge of her violin, we see a woman in the throes of a love affair, a grand passion so complete and un-restrained that we even watch her implode in the ecstasy of orgasm.

BABE BOOSTER
Enhance your sensuality with the elements: fire, earth, air, water. Light scented candles, feed each ot her fruit, mimic the pattern of each other's breathing, sip wine from a shared goblet.

I don't mean that Nadja necessarily feels the rising tides of sensation in her pelvis. I mean that her erotic sense is so fully engaged as she transforms a bow and four strings into an unearthly choir that, as she lures the music to a shattering peak, she radiates rapture. She becomes the essence of eroti-cism, and it is the music that is her lover. Nadja culls creativity from her erotic core—expelling art through a physicality as well tuned as a Stradivarius.

One needn't be a violinist to channel the creative up through the erotic. This is one of the greatest gifts of the erotic sense—the metamorphosis of sensation into art. We block creative energy and sexual energy in the same way—by the same fear of authenticity and of being fully ourselves—and we summon them with our incantations of self-acceptance.

Just as we are taught not to touch ourselves to invoke pleasure, we are taught not to brag about our attributes. Both are equally guilt-ridden pleasures.

A few days ago, I referred to a friend in passing as "a beautiful woman." It was a toss away, the topic really wasn't her at all. So, she confessed later, she bit down on her urge to say, "No, I'm not!" But she felt painted into a corner. If she let my statement pass as her due—sheer vanity! Yet, if she disputed it, she feared making the conversation all about her, plus rudely invalidating my perceptions. Keeping her mouth shut was the lesser evil, pointing out the perversity of our everyday etiquette and their attendant shames. I was so glad she later confessed. She reminded me how much we need to exercise our vanity and our self-acceptance.

This is an exercise in outrageous bragging. I want you to sing from the rooftops your answers to the questions: What have you done for you lately? What qualities have you admired in yourself lately? In what flamboyantly gluttonous ways have you sinned lately?

As if that isn't enough, try this: If you were a new car, gunning your engine as part of a multimillion-dollar ad campaign, what would be said of you? Yes, I realize the automobile is viewed as a masculine metaphor. It is also a power metaphor, so no shirking this now!

Write that description of you, V8 engine and all shiny new. Then read it out loud. Read it to yourself in the mirror. Really look at yourself!

See if you can get your best gal pal to do this exercise with you. Trade places. Write an ad campaign for one another, then exchange pages and read aloud the one your friend wrote for you and vice versa. You'll learn a lot about each other and yourselves that way.

The Erotic Is a Direct Source of Artistic Inspiration

Today women are making sexual art, poetry, theatre, and performance in honor of their own and other women's erotic experiences, and this art, in turn, is waking others from erotic slumber.

Visual artists' work adorns the walls of galleries and cafes in cities across the country, each making lucent statements about woman's experience. Guerilla artists stake out their territory on the Internet, taking on lust, oppression, and political domination.

The erotic muse is alive in the language of women's hip-hop, where *bitch*, *ho*, and *cunt* are power words, not slams. The muse is alive in "clit lit," as women spin tales about their sensitive pearl, engorged and enshrined. Women are painting, drawing, constructing their truths, reaching a handful, reaching millions—as Eve Ensler has in her *Vagina Monologues*.

Sex workers get in on the act proudly. Here in Seattle where I live, the annual Fallen Women Follies dazzles audiences with performers ranging from virtuoso to obscenely comical, energized by the sexy narrative of their lives.

Have you ever wondered why the artist throughout history has been the sexual bohemian? Why the most iconoclastic thinkers are the most innovative in their sexual lives—and why we're so fascinated with such individuals as Pablo Picasso, Jackson Pollack, Frida Kahlo, Anaïs Nin, and Henry Miller, to name just a handful. Is it that we are captivated with the sex lives of everyone public, or is it something more? Perhaps we know intuitively that creativity and eroticism are inescapably intertwined—the real double helix that wickedly animates us, rather than simply bestows life.

The Erotic Motivates Sexual Boldness and Authenticity

College women today are "hooking up" easily but demanding pleasure rarely. Research tells us that, like their mothers, they actively assert their needs only under special conditions, such as when they're in love. They masturbate infrequently and do not have regular orgasms with partners. All too conscious of craving love and connection but out of touch with their eroticism, they supply men with the pleasures they hesitate to take for themselves. They're collecting experiences that they'll probably look back on in ten years as informative and broadening, but not much more. And they deserve more. You deserve more.

In discovering how deep the buried streams of your eroticism run, you can no longer silently ignore your needs. You'll become bold in choreographing your sexual experiences and inviting your lovers to explore your mysteries: *let me show you how…touch me here, like this…yes…oh yes!* Classes in erotic boldness are not taught at universities, but a Babe bares her appetites and acts on the radical desire to fill them. She dedicates herself to becoming her own best teacher.

Choose a day when you are free to design your own schedule. From the moment you open your eyes until you close them sixteen hours later, you will commune with the forces of pleasure. Surround yourself with beauty and fragrance, dedicate your body to erotic sensation, and focus on the salaciously sexual. As you move through the day, ask yourself over and over: *What would please me right now?*

Your Erotic Pleasure Trip begins as you bring each of your senses to life. In the morning, stretch and touch yourself intimately before you even think about rolling out of bed. Bathe instead of shower, massage your skin with fragrant oils, and apply your makeup and style your hair as if you have a date with someone very special. You do, actually—yourself. Dress as if for an assignation—silky underthings that caress your skin—soft, textured, sexy clothing. And jewelry. You want to sparkle today.

At breakfast, treat yourself to a mimosa. A caviar omelet. Throughout the day, create opportunities to delight your senses. Let the strains of music follow you every-where. Buy Casablanca lilies for your desk, call your lover at work and tell him you're touching yourself slowly as you speak—and do it.

Stroll in the park or arboretum, read poetry, touch your breasts in your car, and let the driver of the diesel in the next lane catch you. Speak to a beautiful stranger and think about your pussy as you talk of the weather. Practice walking like a god-dess. Practice leading with your pelvis and walking like a slut. Squeeze your pelvic muscles often. Dance—shimmy and twirl to the music in your heart.

Drink lots of water floating with berries or lime. Shop for a new sex toy. Browse a small bookstore and page through gorgeous books of erotic photography. Take yourself to lunch, alone, at the most beautiful restaurant in town. Go shopping at a men's store and flirt with the salesmen. Fantasize about taking one, two, all of them into the dressing rooms!

Have a massage. Buy rich chocolate truffles but don't eat them all at once. Savor one now. Make yourself wait for another because you want to *tease*, not deprive. Sit in the sun and feel its warmth on your face. Taste the breeze.

This is *your* day. Include erotic and sensual gifts that will cast their private spell on you. Push exquisite excess to the limits of your endurance. Can you allow your-self this one day—just one—of complete self-absorption? I think you can. And that means you can bring any part of this day—even just a tiny slice of it—to *every* day. This is how you become attuned to your erotic sense: by bringing it to life as a nuanced facet of your everyday world.

The Erotic Challenges the Language of Power

The language of power is male. Words and ideas that appear to be universal often reflect a male-oriented window on the world. We call this vision phallocentric—quite literally, centered on the penis. In a phallocentric universe, having sex means intercourse. Genitalia meeting genitalia, that alone is sex. Ask Bill Clinton.

But are penetration and *his* orgasm sex for a woman? Of course not. Every woman knows that, so why is it still a matter of hot debate? In a female-centered world, having sex would mean having your breasts stroked, your thighs caressed, your clit licked, your G-spot stimulated, your feet massaged. A penis might or might not be involved. It would mean kissing until you feel faint. It would mean orgasms of the soul and spirit as well as of the body. It would mean mind-blowing, heart-stopping, ecstatic sexual sensation with no pressure to orgasm at all.

The misguided notion that women want intimacy more than sex may come from the fact that women haven't had enough pleasure to realize they want more. To feel the press of desire, we must yearn for a rapture we know is within reach. As we delve into the erotic, the whole meaning of *having sex* changes, and the meaning of having great sex changes even more. The world, instead of being processed through the "mind" of the penis, is reconfigured through the whole-body eroticism of the goddess sex. Think back to my experience in Maine. Did I have sex? From a phallocentric point of view, no. But from a whole-body, woman-centered point of view, maybe I had sex with the wind.

Erotic energy for women is spiral energy that swirls through us in a windswept way. We reach crests and draw back from them, we orgasm and immediately become aroused and ready to be taken to further erotic heights. We can climax from kissing, from having our breasts stimulated, from thinking intense sexual thoughts without being touched at all. We can come in our dreams. For women, the erotic sense is the winding, circling, carousel of sensation. We are curves and circles and spirals dancing. As Inga Muscio, the author of *Cunt*, writes:

Sexual expression is a current of kinetic energy running through our bodies. It whirligigs up our cunts, charges through our entire being and slam dances on out into the world back through our cunts.

Whirligig! Which reminds me, I don't particularly care for the phrase "having sex." I admit, I use it, but I don't really like it much because it's act-oriented, male-oriented, and cock-oriented—not whirligiggy. Besides, who is being "had" anyway? And isn't it a bit too much like having Chinese for Sunday dinner or having a headache?

I prefer to turn sex into a verb. To sex. *To sex like a goddess. She would sex every night if she could.* They get together to sex. The verb "to sex" is better than "to screw" or "have sex" because it is inclusive of all forms of sexual expression. Mouths doing all that mouths do can be sexing. Lying in each others arms and stroking one another intimately can be sexing. When we change the language to suit our needs as women, we reframe the entire discussion about sexuality.

Let's reconsider the ways we conform our language to fit the dominant culture and allow our words to express our own uniquely feminine experience instead. In this way, we rescue ourselves from what sex revolutionary Susie Bright calls "vocabulary bondage." Once we consider how we speak, we have to ask the next obvious question. Why don't we have language for the pleasure points in our body that glides off our tongues with the ease of their colors, like ruby, or fuschia, or rose? To brandish these words is to be grounded in our feminine power. Inga Muscio found her own path to power in *Cunt*. Although it may not be your path or your ideal choice of words, it is worth reflecting upon. She writes:

> *There are not many things which unite all women. I have found "cunt," the word and the anatomical jewel, to be a venerable ally in my war against my own oppression. Besides global subjugation our cunts are the only common denominator I can think of that all women irrefutably share. We are divided from the word. We are divided from the anatomical jewel. I seek reconciliation.*

In her book *Full Exposure*, Susie Bright penned one of my favorite lines: "Erotic experience is a wake-up call; it's the sign that you're not only alive, you're bursting."

Erotic pleasure is an elixir we can sip like wine. It can be our antidote to depression, to fear, to shame. Yet, it's no news by now that some women fear this pleasure. Before any of us can savor our own erotic potions, we must feel entitled. Certainly, a Babe feels entitled to love wisely, to speak up, to feel joy, to sex!

To the extent that your eroticism is part of the free exchange of energies flowing through your every pore and cell, then the distinction among sensual pleasure, sexual pleasure, and erotic feeling are blurred a dozen times a day. As your awareness of that delicious blur grows, you'll feel joy and power in the smallest detail of your sensation-loaded life.

EXERCISE Take your Whatchamacalit for a Ride

Think about the pink flower between your legs, richer with nerve endings per millimeter than any other part of the human body. Can you happily speak of it using language that doesn't sound like it leaped from a medical text? When you wish to make reference to "that part," what do you say? Can you say the word in conversation as easily as you can in bed? Can you say it as comfortably as you can say "breast" or "butt" or "toe"? Let's take the language for a ride:

Say each of these words out loud:

muff	cooch	heater	snatch	cuny	cunny	pleasure pie
pussty	vutlva	crotch	cunt	coochie	punany	

Choose one that you especially like—or by all means come up with your own—and some time within the next forty-eight hours, take it for a conversational test-drive by using it without hesitating, apologizing, or explaining. You don't get your Babe diploma until you can do this with ease!

You're thinking, of course, how do I work the conversation around so I can use one of those words in the first place? Aha! That's half the test, Babe.

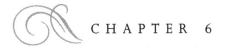

CHAPTER 6

Kindling Erotic Fantasy

Stroke your sexual flame with scintillating stories

IN THE EARLY nineties, I hosted a television series called *Playboy's Secret Confessions and Fantasies.* The series was based on actual people's sexual fantasies and true confessions filmed (using actors) as artful, sexy vignettes.

A typical episode looked like this: I'd start by introducing a five- or six-minute erotic film depicting a sexual fantasy or confession brought to life. Afterward, I'd interview the story's originator and we'd discuss the circumstances surrounding the confession or the meaning of the fantasy, that is, if it actually meant anything at all! Each show contained two film sequences and two interviews.

During pre-production, we were faced with the obvious problem of finding seventy-two people for the thirty-six episodes whose stories were both suitable for filming and who were able to talk about their feelings on air. And yes, they had to "look good," since this was, after all, the Playboy Channel! As producers, we had to kiss a lot of frogs (storywise) to find so many princes and princesses. Not everyone with a scintillating fantasy could express themselves well in conversation, and not everyone who was articulate had a particularly unique story to share. And then, to add to the equation, there was that pesky attractiveness factor to contend with, which was eventually solved by replacing story originators with actors. (Don't let anyone tell you that reality television is real!)

To find our story sources, we placed ads in newspapers throughout the Los Angeles area—from the *Hollywood Reporter* to the *LA Weekly* to the *Los Angeles Times*—and soon, to my surprise, our offices were swamped with potential confessors eager to reveal their most lurid sexual secrets.

For three months I spent twelve hours a day in a little room with a video camera rolling, interviewing one volunteer after another. Sometimes, drawing the sensational details from my subjects felt a bit like the painstaking extraction of an infected molar. At other times, it was all I could do to pry the subject out of his chair so we could move on to the next in line.

As a result of this rather unusual sidebar to my career, I do believe I've explored face to face and in detail a variation on every fantasy theme imaginable. Even after three hundred or so interviews, some especially poignant, or funny, or just plain weird moments stand out, like the frumpy Van Nuys housewife who fantasized being kidnapped by tribal peoples in Africa who mistake her for the embodiment of their fertility goddess. At first terrified, she soon learns that her function as goddess-figure is to make love with the male in each couple who wishes to conceive. Through his consort with her, his female partner's conception is assured.

And I'll never forget the great-grandmother who showed up with her spanking aficionado magazines in hand, and spoke lovingly of paddling the tight, round bottoms of athletic young men. This aspect of my sexology training, while unusual, was certainly useful. To this day, nothing shocks me. Actually, I'm overjoyed when something merely surprises me!

In spite of the humor with which I look back upon those months, there is no diminishing the remarkable honesty and bravery of those who came to us, willing to bare their souls to strangers in ways they may never have done with intimates. The longing to reveal their stories, to be absolved, perhaps, in the glare of the spotlight, was perhaps the most profoundly real secret behind *Secret Confessions and Fantasies*. Our entire production team was aware of holding something quite precious in their hands. These men and women were offering us nothing less than their demons and their dreams, their hearts in search of healing. In those moments of naked self-revelation we were given enormous power. We held their vulnerability and their precarious confidence, and we took that charge quite seriously.

Why would hundreds of people be so eager to share their souls with strangers? I believe the reason lies with the power of fantasy itself, these extravagant theatrics launched from deep within our erotic cores that cry, "I am sexually alive and will not be contained!" Giving sway to our fantasies unites us with ourselves, and sharing them allows us to be seen and heard at the most elemental level of being.

Sadly, many women fear their fantasies. They worry that their imaginings are sick, perverse. Married women often wonder if having fantasies about others is infidelity. Single straight women worry about lesbian fantasies, while lesbians worry that the presence of men in their fantasies is a betrayal. Some women have told me that when they begin to fantasize, they envision minions of invisible ancestors shaking their index fingers in horror over the wicked, wicked thoughts that just won't go away. Yet, it is in just this delightful wickedness that we seed the endlessly riveting reinvention of ourselves. We crave fantasy as we need dreams in the night. Lost in the wakened trance of our most enthralling sexual imagery, we traverse what author Sally Tisdale calls "the land of the not-done and the wished-for," where we come closest to touching the truth of our inner life. Paired with its intimate collaborator, self-pleasuring, fantasy takes us into a dimension where total exposure, first to ourselves, then perhaps to others, becomes an act of irreproachable power. In fantasy we are bold, we are authentic, we are truly Babes.

Fantasy is our flight school. We may never act on many of the scenes that wend their way through our minds, but should we choose to take a fantasy for a spin, we have already enjoyed practice runs that transform the exotic into the near-familiar, and the fearful into the thrilling.

No matter how sexually adventurous we think we are, in the realm of fantasy we can be far more daring. And no matter how comfortable with fantasy we attempt to be, the real test of our willingness to expand is in journeying toward the forbidden (whatever "forbidden" means to each of us). In fantasy, we travel the world without cost or consequence. If we choose to constrain ourselves, we are serving the devils of deprivation, not the goddess of pleasure.

The Abominable Normal

Women so often ask me if a particular sort of fantasy is "normal" that I have come to think of the word itself as an abomination. Imbedded beliefs about normalcy can keep very juicy and inspiring fantasies at bay, and very juicy and inspired Babes under control.

Tell me, what do you think of this fantasy. Is it normal?

You daydream that you're at the movies, sitting between two male strangers. You unbutton your jacket to reveal bare breasts in the half-light. One stranger looks, the other one pretends not to notice. You stroke yourself, your nipples harden, long and hard, and very visible. The film is no longer that interesting for one stranger. He stares at you instead. You smile, and his hand comes to rest on your thigh, so you shift, your miniskirt riding up until he feels your crotch, also bare, even your muff, which is hot, moist and shaven, soft as a baby's skin. His eyebrows raise a notch. The guy on the other side can't resist a peek at you with this utter stranger fumbling between your legs. He looks straight at your breasts in the other guy's hands, and puts a hand on your left knee. You take it and place his thumb in your mouth. He leans in and replaces it with his tongue. Your mouths are frantic, nibbling, sucking, and now the other one wants a kiss too. You turn to him. Three of his right fingers are up your cunt, which is now dripping and even hotter. You can smell your musk in the flickering darkness. The left guy's hand bumps into the right guy's hand by mistake. They both say "sorry." You laugh. One of them bends and takes a nipple in his mouth. The other does the same. One reaches into his pants and begins to stroke himself. Whose fingers are in your cunt? Can't tell, but he's good. You come. The lights come up. You get up. You leave. You don't bother to say goodbye.

Normal or not?

Actually, this was a trick question. The only response that matters: Did you find it even a little bit arousing? Did it inspire a fantasy of your own? What did you like about it? What would you improve upon?

Just for fun, stop reading for a moment and consider the basic scenario sketched above. You are sitting in a movie theater between two strangers. What happens? Close your eyes and imagine this set up. How does the drama unfold? (Consider this an instructive "intermission.")

Guiltless Pleasures

Fantasy may be the only place in your own personal universe where you have complete permission to be an artist of the avant garde. The dreamy images and sensations alive in fantasy are the tools of your creative expression. What self-respecting artist asks whether her imagery is normal? Who asks whether it fits neatly into a statistical average or comes close to a numerical mean? Any true artist would be appalled to hear her work described as creatively average. Fantasy is no place to search for normalcy. It is the dimension in which we look for the extraordinary.

Some therapists suggest that if you are uncomfortable with any of your sexual fantasies—if a fantasy, confessed to any acquaintance would embarrass you or make you feel bad—you should exclude it from your repertoire. Such well-intentioned but poor advice fails to account for the fact that certain politically incorrect fantasies feel shameful precisely because women have been pummeled by attitudes such as these, brainwashed by the idea that only certain fantasy scenarios are acceptable. To suggest that you revise your fantasies simply because they initially make you uncomfortable only succeeds in giving power to such repressive constructs. A Babe does not buy into this foolishness.

Women who have experienced sexual abuse or violence in their lives often find that the hottest fantasy scenarios are those which contain some aspect of the energies bound up in their abuse, such as domination, control, or humiliation. In their fantasies, they submit to others or command power against others, or both. It's understandable that you might wonder and ask whether arousal that appears to be chained to memories of fear and denigration can be healthy. But these are the wrong questions. If you doubt the function of a fantasy, you should be asking:

- Are these fantasies helping me gain control of energies that were once outside my control?
- How do the contradictions in my fantasy help me make peace with my past?

BABE BOOSTER

Fantasies are your friends! Building them into your repertoire will only serve to enhance your sex life. Better yet, sharing them with a lover will turn the heat up a notch!

- Do these fantasies give me something enriching—something for my own pleasure—to take away from the world of pain I once knew?
- How do these fantasies empower me as a sexually alive, consciously erotic woman?

These fantasies came into being to provide a balance of power. Remember, we own our fantasies. We own the set up, the action, and the outcome. We own our desire. It matters not from where that desire springs so long as we lay claim to it as choice-making adults. Besides, fantasies are more than literal representations of desire. They are like dreams carrying symbolic messages. If you fantasize being raped, you may be revealing a hunger to be so desired that someone is willing to breech law and all consideration of civilized behavior to have you. Or you may want to exploit your own unruly impulses and direct your aggression where it can do no harm, at yourself, for your own pleasure. You are rapist and raped, your are abuser and abused.

If any fantasy leaves you wringing wet, exhausted from quivering orgasms yet guilty for the pleasure, instead of replacing the scenario with proper love stories, ask yourself "Why the guilt?" What unacceptable ideas about yourself does the fantasy highlight? What needs burn within you that you believe you're not entitled to possess? Instead of running from those needs, embrace them with added fervor. Desires embraced and understood rarely do harm. Desires drawn underground can be dangerous or at least stultifying. Yet, if you feel your fantasies are tinged with self-hatred or disturbing urges to do real violence to others, your answers to the previous questions should illuminate these issues. A sex therapist can help you work with troublesome fantasies that feel too cumbersome to contain on your own.

BABE BOOSTER

Take your lover on a fantasy field trip—surprise him with an excursion to an erotic film, a sex-toy shop, or a "gentleman's" club.

Joy and Pain

Pleasure is not without its antithesis. Suffering and pleasure are equally strong, compelling forces. Erotically, they are yin and yang, light and dark, and one without the other is devoid of the dynamic tension that produces heightened responses in many of us. In fact, extreme pleasure is in itself a form of suffering. Intense, unremitting pleasure is almost unendurable, it is almost pain. Have you never said to a lover whose touch left you limp as a rag doll and near tears: "Stop, I can't stand anymore (pleasure)," and then you pushed through the pleasure/pain barrier to discover more anyway?

Like pleasure and suffering, our most stirring fantasies juxtapose two opposing themes: The will and the power to act upon another, and the surrender to being acted upon.

Nearly every fantasy is an intricate choreography, intertwining action and surrender, dominance and submission. If you thought those words applied only to "kinky" sex, take note—they apply to all sexual exchanges. In the movie theatre fantasy, the woman was both willful and surrendered. She unbuttoned her jacket and exposed her breasts to two strangers. Willful. She remained impassive while they suckled and penetrated her. Surrendered.

In your own version of that movie theatre fantasy, in what ways did you wield power? In what ways did you surrender to the will of the strangers?

In some fantasies, the balance clearly leans toward one or another edge. Our sense of self in the fantasy is primarily directive, aggressive, dominant, only secondarily receptive, or the other way around, where the power is exchanged in a manner that sends us spiraling into submissive rapture. You may notice that despite the differences in the details, most of your fantasies—or the fantasies that you respond to most strongly when you read them—place you primarily at one end of the act-upon/surrender-to continuum. Or you might discover you are eminently flexible, able to pirouette between poles with agility and grace.

Limiting your exploration of fantasy limits more than your capacity for sexual authenticity—it limits your personal authenticity as well.

How can you know what resonates deep down in your erotic core unless you expose your mind to an array of possibilities? How do you know what touches you unless you allow your imagination to be stroked? How do you know who you really are if you turn away from experiences that reflect your image back to you?

Tristan Rainer, author of *The New Diary*, tells of teaching a women's writing class at the University of California and asking her students to use their diaries to record their sexual experiences. Celebrating erotic experience by describing it in specific detail in their diaries helped her students develop a personal language of sexuality, and recognize the tides and moods of their whimsical erotic cycles. Writing led to a deep respect for the erotic, a moving toward each woman's center. Giving permission to imaginary sexuality seemed to liberate them in other areas of their creative life. One, for instance, cured herself of a writing block that had kept her from finishing any of her other stories. She discovered in herself a fully developed and sophisticated fantasy world that, when written out in her diary, seemed to free her to creatively use the energy that had gone into repressing her fantasies.

If fantasy is creatively evocative, if there is no right or wrong, no healthy or unhealthy fantasy, then what would stop you from exploring an unlimited repertoire of fantasy and lay bare the most alluring for repeated use? Usually, it is a fear of these possibilities:

1. Your inner critic's horrified judgment (for example, saying to yourself, "You are so sick to be turned on by *that*!");
2. Your yearning for something that, if acted upon, would surely get you into trouble (for example, lead to your behaving like a slut!).

Put another way, we fear fantasy because we have not yet learned to trust ourselves—to trust ourselves to accept ourselves in all our diversity, to trust ourselves to take responsible action on our desires.

Limiting your fantasies because you don't trust yourself is tantamount to treating yourself like a child who needs to be protected from the big bad world. How very unBabelike!

A Babe Can Eroticize *Everything*

It's impossible to talk about fantasy without bringing up the subject of shame. For women, shame is the tightly cinched bond tied around sex and desire that constricts our lives and our imagination. There are two ways to absolve ourselves of shame. One is to speak of it, share it, expose it to the light and watch it burn away. The other is to use it, to eroticize it. Fantasy allows us to utilize shame in extraordinarily creative ways. If you allow yourself this privilege, you triumph over shame. When you can eroticize everything, turn fear and vulnerability and powerlessness and anxiety into a kind of sexual fantasy game, you are healing your shame and giving yourself permission to access the erotic within you at will. The contradiction inherent in wanting and fearing the same thing is resolved through fantasy.

Mary Beth was raised devoutly Catholic—parochial school, church on Sundays, the works. She eventually left the church, but the church didn't leave her. Its dogma kept her sexuality in check until she learned to exaggerate the very obstacles that stood in her way. Images of stepping into the confessional and being forced to make contrition to the priest entered her fantasies. Instead of falling to her knees with rosary in hand, she'd drop to her knees with Father Mike in hand, in mouth, and every other orifice

> **BABE BOOSTER**
> *Write your hottest fantasy on a Post-it note and slip it into your lover's underwear drawer or briefcase so that he finds it unexpectedly (be prepared for the heat!).*

as well. In other fantasies, she consorted with the devil himself in raging, unholy exhaltation. As she shared and enacted these stories with her partner, dogma and desire found reconciliation, and her shame dissolved.

Darcy's story swerves powerfully in quite the opposite direction. When she was in the tenth grade, she went out with a boy whose mouth was bigger than any other organ, and their tame back-seat gropings were transformed into rabid back-door pokings as the tale wended its way through the school corridors. Darcy was slimed for the duration of her school years. Even though she grew more bookish and removed from social intercourse with each passing year, the slut label and the shame stuck. By senior year, Darcy stopped trying to fight her reputation, "Why not screw around? I was taking the rap anyway," she concluded. But her escapades felt deadening and after a few months she retreated again. Then, just after graduation, she had a dream: "I was a pleasure goddess in an opulent temple where each grandly appointed chamber was devoted to a unique fantasy theme. I loved guiding my patrons toward the fulfillment of their most coveted sexual desires. This was my calling, and like a priestess of ancient times, I was honored and rewarded in gold and precious stones. I had an actual orgasm in my dream as I was servicing a beautiful young man. It was his first time and we were both overjoyed with the feelings we shared."

In her dream, her unconscious had reframed "slut" as "sacred whore"—which is in itself a powerful feminine archetype. Mysteriously enough, at the time of her dream, Darcy had no previous exposure to this luminous imagery as it appears in history. Yet, from that moment on, Darcy's sexuality began to flower, first in private as she masturbated to variations on her dream, and later, when she met her first real boyfriend and merged her persona as pleasure goddess into her romantic life.

Both Mary Beth and Darcy transformed an obstacle to ecstasy into a transcendent refuge from ordinary life. Mary Beth exaggerated the obstacle itself, building on the concept of sin, plunging more deeply into the dark dimension. Darcy reframed her obstacle, replacing soiled betrayal with service and sacredness—one might say, veering toward the light. Neither approach is healthier or preferable, just different. And both achieved the same effect of reparation and healing.

Based on their stories, you can see the reflection of what Jack Morin, author of *The Erotic Mind*, has dubbed a "core erotic theme" in both Mary Beth and Darcy's fantasy life. Our unique histories produce attractions to certain narratives, which become dominant in our fantasy life or our actual romantic life, transforming old wounds and conflicts into a nucleus of arousal. Women drawn to distant or unavailable men may actually be playing out facets of their core erotic theme. Men excited by emotionally volatile women—same story. That magnetic attraction to the inappropriate or forbidden? A most common expression of core narrative.

Letty, a suburban mom, was confused and disturbed by a persistent fantasy of rape by a gang of young black boys. She was able to accept it when she saw how growing up in a racially mixed neighborhood, with a dad who expressed antipathy toward nonwhites, conferred an unshakable allure upon the dark young men she dared not date. How better to guiltlessly reconcile her conflict than with a fantasy of domination by not one, but many?

Our peak erotic experiences usually encompass some elements of strong attraction coupled with an obstacle to desire. This, according to Morin, is the formula for arousal: Attraction + Obstacles = Excitement. In our everyday lives we usually try to limit the degree to which we introduce serious obstacles. Our fantasy worlds need not know such boundaries.

Pamela harbors fantasies of extreme humiliation—being tied up, whipped, urinated upon, and then forced to remain still as her partner masturbates and comes all over her. Before raising your eyebrows, consider the prohibitive and therefore tempting matter of exchanging body fluids. Doesn't that add another dimension to Pamela's fantasy, softening what might have seemed "way out there" at first blush? Actually, humiliation fantasies among both women and men are relatively common, and we are more likely to judge them in others when we are shamed by them in ourselves. However, if we remember that our core erotic themes are imposed by the unique challenges of living and loving in each of our lives, the inclusion of degrading fantasies makes sense. Like shame, experiences of humiliation and debasement are ubiquitous in childhood and adolescence. As we eroticize rather than repress them, we snatch back their power for ourselves.

EXERCISE Exploring Your Fantasy Secrets

In your journal complete the following exercises:

1. Describe a sexual fantasy you've always wanted to enact but have not had the opportunity to play out yet.

2. Describe a sexual fantasy you find extremely exciting but would probably be unwilling to disclose to anyone—even a lover. However, you might consider living out this fantasy with a stranger if none of your friends or partners knew.

3. Describe a sexual fantasy you find extremely exciting, would probably be willing to disclose to a lover, but would not enact.

4. Describe a sexual fantasy you would not do and would probably not reveal even to a lover.

5. Describe a sexual fantasy you know for sure you would never tell anyone— ever, ever, ever—and would certainly never do.

6. Now imagine that you have a lover who tells you his or her most private, never before divulged fantasy. And imagine that his fantasy is the same as, and complementary to, item five, the one you said you'd never, ever tell. (By complementary, I mean that whatever he says he would like to do to a partner is exactly what you fantasize having done to you, or vice versa.) What would you do now? Would his revelation change the way you feel about disclosing your fantasy? Would the meaning of "never, ever do" change?

Playing With Fire

In my work I've come across and written about what I call the danger-fear-excitement connection, a kind of first cousin to Morin's later observations about the combustion that occurs when attraction meets obstacles. Is there any greater obstacle than real danger, real fear?

Some women are sexual daredevils who thrive on moments of reckless abandon, where true danger is the aphrodisiac. Others do so only in fantasy. Barrie, for example, fantasizes driving cross-country, stopping in small towns, sexing it up with one or two of the locals, and then tipping her hat and driving away—a kind of modern day, femme version of the restless cowboy traveling Route 66. It isn't just the freedom that drives Barrie's fantasy—it's the danger, the anonymity, and the power of numbers.

Courtney shares Barrie's fantasy, only she has lived a good piece of it. An attraction to reckless power and the suspense of the unknown took her from Santa Fe to Savannah, sexing her way across the nation.

As Barrie imagines, and Courtney knows so well, playing with fire *always* opens us up to the possibility of getting burned. Even if the fire is a string of lovers behind your husband's back, the thrill comes from riding an exhilarating wave of fear between the commission of an act and the moment when you either come face to face with its consequences or realize that you've escaped them. Whatever danger you dabble in, from the instant you first contemplate the act, the burning question is this: Will you get away with it—or won't you? The more partners you have, the more uncontrollable they are, the more there is to lose, the more scared you get, the more exciting the encounter can seem.

The relationship between danger, fear, and excitement is documented at the biological level, and the sexiness of fear is well known as it relates to soldiers in battle, who have written copiously of becoming sexually aroused during or after an especially dangerous mission. Athletes report a sexual thrill in daredevil sports. Even our language patterns allude to a fundamental connection between fear and sexual excitement. Skiers, for example, often describe perilous jumps as orgasmic experiences. And the term *risk* is actually rooted in the French word *risqué*. Risky sex in public places is a favorite means of spicing up a tired sex life. Bare-backing (anal sex without protection) is known in the gay community as a secret thrill. The sexiness of fear also partially explains the appeal that the "bad boy" holds for so many women, whether in real life or in fantasy. Such partners seem sexier because they are socially less acceptable, and perhaps genuinely dangerous. Just think of all the women out there writing to guys in prison. It sure isn't because they can take them to the nicest places. For women who deep down fear the defiant aspects of themselves, getting it on—even if just via e-mail—with men who symbolize insurgency is as close to being a Babe as they're willing to get.

Poet Rosemary Daniell used to fit the profile of the woman who sought adventure through her choice of men. At once the embodiment of cloistered Southern womanhood and the raunchy renegade who strained to escape the "prison of the bourgeois" in which she was raised, Rosemary found excitement in the arms of men who lived dangerously, drank too much, and often exhibited a violent form of male chauvinism. She even wrote a book, *Sleeping with Soldiers: In Search of the Macho Man*, chronicling her sexual odyssey among modern-day swashbucklers—soldiers of fortune, oil riggers, paratroopers, contemporary cowboys—whose macho was exaggerated almost to the point of caricature.

In the grip of lovers who acted out her secret wildness and hidden desires for anarchy, Rosemary could reconcile her drive for danger and excitement with her need to remain appropriately feminine. As she put it, "The more macho the man, the more traditionally feminine—passive and virtuous—I felt." She never experienced anxiety about sex roles with a man who was a Real Man, for she was certain of his masculinity and, thus, her femininity.

Rosemary's adventures had their costs. She told me of a number of incidents in which the men she picked up became threatening. She believes that she survived without getting hurt by relying on her abundant Southern charm. For example, Rosemary told me this tale:

"I was spending some time up in the Georgia Mountains. I picked up a very good-looking, husky guy, about 250 pounds, and took him back to the cabin—there was nothing around for miles. He was high on Valium, so he had trouble performing sexually and we just went to sleep. The next morning, the snow was falling outside, and we just lay in bed watching it when he turned to me and said, 'You know those women in the next county that were raped and murdered? Well, I'm the one who did it.' "I laughed, and pretended he was just kidding. I tried to act real cool, real casual, but I was scared. When I got up to get dressed I remember standing with my back to him, putting my sweater over my head—and he suddenly came up behind me and put his big forearm around my neck. I quickly leaned into him, all lovey-dovey, as if he was just being affectionate, and I told him I had to hurry and dress because someone was going to be here any second to take me to breakfast. A little while later, thank goodness, a Jeep did pull up...."

Rosemary's story goes back quite a few years. Today she's in touch with her own power so she doesn't need to borrow it from macho men or make any man a metaphor for the adventure-loving part of herself. Rosemary has become quite the Babe. But her fantasies-come-to-life remind me that danger is one matter in the wakened trances we explore in our bedrooms—alone or with a trusted lover—and quite another out in the world where daredevil sex can sometimes translate into taking fool-hardy chances. I'm hardly one to tell a Babe which risks are healthy and which are too extreme; I can only suggest that you pay close attention to your own instincts and protect your renegade spirit so that when playing with fire you won't go up in flames.

Cultivating Your Fantasy Life

In the interest of discovering more about the range of fantasy that excites you, you're about to read four distinctly different stories. These are the genuine articles, written by four different women, reflecting their authentic fantasy lives. These women are truly Babes for being brave enough to lend their intimate writing for your pleasure.

As you read, I'd like you to try to suspend all critical thought and allow the images to tease you. Remember, these are not descriptions of sexual scenarios you are being asked to enact, they are simply mind candy, meant to arouse your curiosity, to turn up your heat.

Before you begin, you might want to make sure you won't be interrupted. Get real comfy, turn on some soft music, and relax as you read these short tales.

THE OTHER MAN

The party was perfect. The house was large and the rooms rambling, crowded with people enjoying an abundance of food and drink. He moved through the masses, deliberately avoiding conversation, getting by with a nod or a quick wave for those he recognized. She followed close behind him, her eyes cast down. She knew she was behaving splendidly tonight, dressed perfectly for his agenda. Wearing no bra as instructed, her knob nipples were rock hard, sticking out defiantly against her crepe blouse. Her tight skirt flared slightly at the hemline just above her knees and she wore nothing beneath it. She knew he enjoyed the admiring glances other men bestowed on her, and it made him hot to wonder how quickly those admirers could be urged to run a hand under her skirt, tracing her silky thighs to the wet spot. Did they know what could happen, she wondered, did they see his attitude and her subservience to him?

They entered a room that was not too full; only a few clusters of men stood in conversation, a perfect setting. He found a place where they could sit at a ninety degree angle to one another, knees almost touching. He sat down first, as always, leaning back, legs planted firmly, hands clasped behind his head, relaxed. She waited, eyes only on him, until he was totally comfortable, then sat down slowly. Once she was seated she knew she should open her legs immediately, but perversely she didn't. That would cost her later, she smiled inside. He stared at her intently until she slowly parted her knees. He didn't release her from his penetrating gaze until her legs were where he wanted them—thighs ten inches apart. Not an obviously unladylike posture, but any alert observer would see that she was purposefully opening up to him.

He engaged her in casual conversation, comments about the food, the party, peppered with graphic, sometimes crude remarks about her delightful body, in particular her private parts, always so far from private in his presence. Her face flushed with sexual excitement. He knew her. He knew how she felt right now, thrilled by his words and references, yet slightly uncomfortable holding her thighs open and keeping her body available and perfectly still. It took great restraint for her to rivet her attention on him, to resist the temptation to look for the reactions of others to their tableau.

He leaned over to her now, wooing her with romantic expressions and explicit descriptions of what he would be doing to her breasts, nipples, thighs, and her cunt. At the same time he scanned the rest of the room looking for the right man.

She knew he spotted him by the shift in his expression, the set of his jaw. Someone was making no attempt to disguise his interest in her body or the way it was being controlled. She shivered, excited, nervous, too. He was touching her knees gently, grazing them with his fingertips, and asking her if she wanted them inside her cunt lips. She flushed in answer. No matter how many times he had said these things to her, she would always flush, which embarrassed her and excited him tremendously. She could feel someone else near her now, but didn't dare try to sneak a better look.

She could see the bulge in his pants growing, his cock beginning to stiffen. Without hesitation he moved his right hand slowly, deliberately, up her skirt between her open knees, stroking her inner thighs. Then, with his eyes focused somewhere behind her, he slipped his fingertips between her fat, full cunt lips, right into her juicy honeypot and stroked away. She sighed and leaned back, not caring about her appearance. Her head tilted almost imperceptibly in the direction of his gaze but he grasped her chin, rooting her attention firmly where it belonged. His eyes held hers, then veered away again as he ran his fingers up and down her wet slit, stopping to tweak her swollen clit. Surely the stranger would be touching himself, or leaning against a side table, moving his crotch across the edge.

Holding his breath, his cock throbbing hard against his zipper, he rammed his fingers deeper into her cunt, held them still for a moment, pressing hard against her G-spot, then his eyes locked with hers.

He pulled his hand down and away from her thighs quickly. She gasped at the sudden emptiness. He stood up, picked up his drink, and she followed him as they moved smoothly toward the door. He did not look back for a moment, and of course she remained behind him, with her eyes only on him.

THE BIRTHDAY PRESENT

For Alexis' thirtieth birthday her husband brought home a very special present. Her name was Kat, and Kat had a special gift for Alexis, too. Kat's gift was seven inches long, made of hard rubber, and Kat would be wearing her present on a belt that cinched around her hips, that is, when Kat was good and ready. Kat wouldn't let Alexis play with her special present right away. For what seemed like hours to Alexis, Kat insisted on warming Alexis up with mouth and fingers prodding everywhere, driving Alexis into a near convulsive state of desire. All the while, Alexis tried to cajole Kat into doing the one thing she wanted the most. But as the night wore on, if Alexis learned anything, it was that the more she tried to pressure Kat, the more enjoyment Kat got from resisting and teasing. Finally—*finally*—while Alexis was pouring the two of them a glass of wine at the dining room table, Kat came up behind her and wrapped her arms around Alexis' waist. Alexis leaned back into her and felt the tip of Kat's "gift." She set down the wine glasses as Kat's faux-cock slid down her rear cleft and pressed against her little pink hole. Alexis' muscles tightened and she didn't dare move—she barely breathed. She so wanted to feel the surge of Kat's hardness inside of her, and she didn't want to make a single move that would give Kat a reason to tease her any longer.

"Relax now," said Kat, pressing forward so that Alexis had to bend over the sturdy wooden dining room table. She could feel Kat's fingers, thick with warm lube, brush against her bottom hole, and then Kat's cock pushed against her tight opening. Alexis gasped and a cry escaped her as she felt Kat hold her more firmly and push harder against her hips. The thick dick prodded Alexis' anal throat open, and she hungrily took it all inside. The sensation was shockingly wonderful. Kat began to move, finding a rhythm that with each stroke gave Alexis mounting pleasure. Alexis attempted to suck the dildo in deeper, deeper, up to its absolute base. In response, Kat increased the length of her strokes and she reached an arm around Alexis' hips to catch her clitoris with her fingertips. Kat was driving the full length of her shaft in and out of Alexis' ass, electrifying Alexis' whole body. Alexis couldn't separate the fierce pleasure she was receiving from Kat's hard cock from the bliss of Kat's fingers on her clitoris. It all melted into the most exquisite warm throbbing sensation and she lost herself in it, moaning and crying.

Suddenly Kat pulled out of Alexis and turned her over on her back. She quickly, expertly, changed condoms and almost before Alexis knew what was happening, Kat started a slow, easy grind into her pussy. Kat couldn't know it, but she was doing what Alexis liked best—teasing her opening with the head of her cock, then plunging in for long, full thrusts. Damn she's good, Alexis thought. She arched her back and felt the weight of Kat's body rhythmically pushing her to ecstasy. Her moans were growing louder as her whole body pulsated with pleasure. Kat saw Alexis bite her bottom lip as her breathing became more guttural and deep. Kat's fingertips kept tune with her thrusts, playing Alexis' clit like an instrument on every backward motion of her hips. "Oh Kat, kiss me, I'm going to come now," she cried. Kat's mouth covered hers and Alexis felt the full weight of Kat's hips pin her to the table. Alexis exploded, pinwheels of light filling her vision. Oh, it was good, so very good. And then Alexis's husband, who had been watching all along, was there, too, and his mouth met hers and Kat's hungrily.

It was one very happy thirtieth birthday!

LOVE'S SURRENDER

We have been apart so long, Armand and I, and finally, we meet again in his hotel. I leap into the bed where he lies naked. His eyes sparkle, bright and open and inviting me inside, to that place of pleasure and connection we know so very well.

I feel his warmth, peering back into his brown, creamy eyes, and wait for him to beckon. He moves toward my face and his mouth and mine meet, blended, forged into an energy of oneness. I feel his tongue probing and forming an electrical charge with mine. We merge, mouth into mouth, ego past ego, our bodies flowing in synchronous motion like dolphins undulating in the belly of a calm sea. Hands touch hands and ecstasy begins anew with each searing kiss, wet and deep and strong, currents like an ocean engulfing us now.

In the ooze of our loving I feel his penis pressing against me. Armand rolls on top of me, the feel of his hardness sends shock waves into my groin. My body rises up to meet him as I ache for his penis to be inside of me. I feel how wet I am, an ocean of longing welling up to take him diving. He pushes harder, lifts his body, and without losing a beat, he plunges his flame into my ocean. Deep, deep he penetrates the core of my being. We are melting into a union of intense pleasure. I feel the edges of the universe gone now, and oneness is all there is.

Armand thrusts in and out with tender push and pull. Then mightily he throbs up and down the vaginal canal until he is about to reach my cervix. I feel that moment which happens so rarely, when the upper part of my vagina opens the gate. The gate to the Goddess. The gate to bliss. The gate to real union. He has found it once more, and we are off to the highest places we can know as lovers.

"You have passed the gate, my love…" I half speak to him as I contain him, all the way into my essence.

He begins to talk to me, in a soft masculine voice. "Surrender to me, my love. Let me take all of you—come to me, all of you—be all mine. I want you forever. I've never loved like this before, never want to be apart again, can you trust me, *cherie?* I cannot live without you anymore. Say, yes, and I am yours, whatever it takes—let me show you what total surrender into love can be. Oh, I love you, with all my being…."

His words are like magnets, pulling me deeper into him. As I listen, I repeat back sayings and promises, and float into his fantasy as never before. I surrender my body, my words, my heart, my spirit, yes, even my soul, as we travel beyond form, time, and space.

What seem like hours pass, we transcend our orgasms, nine or ten each, repeating the patterns of loving over and over. Then, finally, we share giggles, look into each other's eyes, wet from the tears that such closeness provokes, roll over, and fall asleep.

THE BOY-TOY

Ariana loved the sound the leather made as she glided off the seat of her 1200 Sporty. The ride, the air, the freedom—no one could tie her down.

It was always the same when she walked into the bar—those men thinking they looked so tough in their leather and Harley Davidson gear. Well, they should only know what she knew about what they liked.

The usual greetings were exchanged with the regular crowd, but her attention drifted to the corner of the bar. Seated alone was a tall, broad-shouldered man with the rough good looks that come with riding a bike in all sorts of weather. Perfect for the pleasure she loved so much. She was cold from the ride, but inside the heat was beginning to rise, and she could feel it start spilling from between her legs. She caught his eye for a second and he veered away, but she would not. He glanced again and she half smiled, half sighed. She knew she had him.

She walked over, knowing he would mentally undress her, focusing on her large breasts and ample hips. Her legs were long, emphasized by the knee-high black leather studded boots she wore.

"Haven't seen you here before," she said. "I would have remembered such a potential boy-toy." He wasn't sure how to take that comment. Brazenly, she touched his thigh and squeezed.

"Ah, all muscle." She reached for his groin; he was already growing hard in her hand. He took her move as an invitation, and went for her crotch, but she quickly grabbed his hand. "Oh no, not so fast! I've had a long ride. I need to use the ladies' room." He watched her get up, filled with anticipation.

Five minutes passed, and he couldn't wait. He walked over to the bathroom and knocked. "Baby, come on in." He entered and she grabbed him by the hair, taking him by complete surprise, and kissed him deeply.

Quickly, she unclasped the necklace she wore, a leather c-ring collar, and carefully placed it around his neck, adjusting it to fit him tightly. He offered no resistance.

"You want this?" she said, and opened her blouse, exposing her breasts, placing her hands firmly on her dark pink, erect nipples. He nodded.

"Lock the door."

"Sure, baby."

"No, you little slut, it's Mistress to you! We know who's in control here, don't we?" she commanded, grabbing him by the collar and pressing up against him.

"You, Mistress…and enjoying every minute of it," he said, lightly. She realized he still didn't get that this was no half-hearted game. She drew a pair of handcuffs from her pants pocket. "Now, turn around!"

He did as he was told, and she clamped the cuffs shut. He smiled. "Wipe that silly grin off your face! You're nothing but a little slut here for my amusement! Get down on your knees, and clean up the wet spot I'm standing in on this bathroom floor!"

Although, he started to protest, Ariana gave him a nudge with her boot and he did as he'd been told. Watching him obey made her wetter and wetter, the moisture gushing from inside her as her breathing came in short little gasps.

"You know, I just realized, we haven't named you yet. What's your real name, slave?"

"It's Michael, Mistress."

"Okay, Michele. Michele it's going to be. So listen up, Michele, I'm going to strip you. Can you handle that?"

Michele assented, and in seconds he was naked as a baby. Ariana stroked his broad shoulders, his muscular ass and big, firm cock. Then she removed her clothes, except for her see-through panties and boots.

"Start licking like a good boy," she ordered. He attached his lips to the outside of her panties, and she noticed his cock was leaking delicious, sweet pre-cum.

"No, not there, you fool! Start with my boots!"

As instructed, Michele began licking her boots as if he were working her clit, sucking, biting, making her pussy so wet she felt faint. He eased his way up her thighs, and when she couldn't wait another second, she yanked his head to her already soaked panties. "Oh, you are a good slave," she said, trying to hold back the climax that was building.

Suddenly she slapped him hard across the face—she couldn't give up this control yet. She had to catch him off balance. He looked stunned.

"Say thank you, you worthless piece of shit!"

"Thank you, Mistress!" His cock became harder and made it's own wet spots on the floor.

"Lick that up too—and who told you to stop sucking, anyway? Don't you dare come until I say you can!"

Michele immediately returned to his job. But a few more minutes were all Ariana could take before letting loose with a spasmodic cry and showering his face with cum. "Now you, you slut! Cum all over yourself!"

And Michele, being such an obedient slave, once again did exactly as he was told.

She removed the cuffs and petted him for a long, long time.

"Do you cum here often?" she laughed, and they embraced tightly, certainly not for the last time.

Once your breathing has returned to normal, try rating each of the fantasies on two scales. First, for arousal value—on a scale of one to five, how hot was each? Five means you were panting, one means you caught a chill. Second, for shock effect—on a scale of one to five, how far outside the box of your usual fantasies did each reside? Five means it was so outside your realm that it made your squirm, but not in a good way. One means it was about as shocking as a Burger King commercial.

Did your ratings hold any surprises? For example, did you notice that the more romantic a story, the more turned on you were? Or did you notice you were far more attracted to a certain form of power exchange—willful or surrendered—than you anticipated? Did certain obstacles or dangers get you going more than others?

If you encountered an unexpected reaction, you might be wondering, "What could this *mean*?"

I suspect it means that areas of erotic inhibition are already unraveling within you, that you're open to greater possibilities for pleasure than you knew!

EXERCISE Your Erotic Theme

Have you noticed a predominant erotic theme in your fantasies? If so, think about what it might feel like to stand up before an audience of men and reveal it. Is the prospect exciting, embarrassing, frightening? What kinds of reactions would you anticipate? Think about sharing with an audience of women. How might that feel? What myths and beliefs about acceptable female sexuality might be contributing to how you imagine being perceived by men and by women?

My intention in this chapter was to give you carte blanche to stretch your fantasy world beyond the confines of its previous borders. In the *Afterplay* section later in this book, you'll find suggested books and Internet sites, which can become your guides to even more uninhibited flights of fancy.

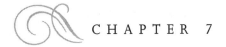

CHAPTER 7

Cultivating Self-Pleasure and Self-Love

Discover your body's sweet spots

W HEN I CAME ACROSS an ancient textbook at a sex therapy conference, my eyes opened wide in shock. Yes, I knew things were bad for women a hundred years ago, just not quite this bad! Check out Professor Prof. Wm. H. Walling's *Sexology*, written in 1904. This is from the chapter *Masturbation, Female*:

> Alas, that such a term is possible! O, that it were as infrequent as it is monstrous, and that no stern necessity compelled us to make the startling disclosures that this chapter must contain! We beseech, in advance, that every young creature into whose hands this book may chance to fall, if she be yet pure and innocent, will at least pass over this chapter, that she may still believe in the general chastity of her sex; that she may not know the depths of degradation into which it is possible to fall.

I don't know about you, but it's way too late for me.

I'm already a fallen woman, abjectly degraded and lovin' it. A Babe is surely the most degraded of creatures. For a Babe, innocence holds no glory and the heinous acts of which the doctor speaks are as natural as breathing.

Yet, the eminent professor Walling might be pleased to know that even now, a hundred years after the publication of his textbook, women are not by and large as enthusiastic about masturbation as the Babe.

Petting the Kitty: Are We Having Fun Yet?

Research on masturbation tells us that there are vast differences between women and men. Not only are more women masturbation "virgins," but among women who do masturbate, we also indulge with far less frequency than the guys.

In early adolescence, when we should be urged to delight in and experiment with our lovely genital flowers, we are instead reminded of the dire consequences of self-stimulation. I think of all the women clients who have shared horror stories about being caught masturbating. One woman's mother even threatened to cut off her fingers. I vividly remember being informed by my mother when I was about eleven that touching myself "down there" would cause a terrible infection. It took me years to see through her fraud. When I learned that boys wanted to touch me down there, too, and the injunctions against giving them access had to do with losing their respect (nice girls don't), I knew that my mom hadn't come clean about the M word. Not all our parents lie outright, but few encourage their daughters to discover the joys of their own womanly flesh. If your mom was more approving of self-pleasure, you are truly among the fortunate.

Think about your own current attitudes toward masturbation. How comfortable are you with the idea of self-pleasure? Jokes such as "at least you don't have to shave your legs for a date with yourself," notwithstanding, how easily do you discuss the topic with friends? Do you share vibrator and other sex toy tips? Could you, like the irrepressible Samantha in *Sex and the City*, march up to the counter at the crowded Sharper Image in midtown Manhattan brandishing your pooped out personal massager and loudly demand that the salesman replace the device that dared to die midstream without so much as a kiss goodbye?

What do you call this private thing you do? Men have so many silly terms for "choking the chicken," and women have so few. Do you Jill-off daily? Based on the letters I receive from men, guys are chronically worried about "beating the meat" too much. "Am I normal to be typing this letter to you, Dr. Joy, with one hand on the keyboard and the other whipping my real joystick?"

When you play with your pearl, do you go after a quick fix or do you gift yourself with luxuriously long sensual sessions? Do you focus only on your clitoris, or do you caress your body—pluck at your breasts, massage your G-spot, employ dildos and other toys to reach into your depths? Do you linger over elaborate fantasies or focus strictly on physical sensation?

Instead of taking for granted your approach to yourself, take a moment to reflect upon your self-seductions. If you were an objective bystander, what would the nature of these excursions tell you about your willingness to cherish your body and savor your capacity for extravagant sexual thrills?

Kathleen, a successful, twenty-nine-year-old lawyer, has a collection of vibrators, which she uses regularly at least once, sometimes two or three times a day. Within minutes she can climax. Her morning orgasm is like a cuppa Joe, charging her up for the courtroom battle of the day. At noon she sometimes sneaks off to the bathroom, pulls her "pocket rocket" from her purse and gives herself a quick energy jolt. At night she treats herself to another session, letting stress bleed away as she comes, and then drifts off to sleep. Kathleen's masturbation is largely what I call "medicinal." Nothing wrong with that, but it tells us a lot about how Kathleen regards her sexuality and her body. Sex is utilitarian. She doesn't pleasure herself with abandon—in fact, she literally abandons herself, tunes herself out, to achieve pleasure.

> **BABE BOOSTER**
>
> *Compose a love letter to yourself.*
> *Begin each day with a one-line love*
> *note. Write it on a napkin in the*
> *coffee shop you frequent or at the*
> *bottom of today's page in your*
> *appointment book.*

Kathleen doesn't like her body much. She makes little time for exercise or self-care. She hates being "fat and flabby" but doesn't change the habits that keep her from being more toned. Kathleen feels that she isn't perfect enough and never will be, so why bother striving for a crown she'll never win? She's good at her job, has lots of girlfriends, and dates often enough to remind herself why she doesn't go out more. ("Men are so demanding and self-centered anyway, who has time for the bull?") She has a shelf filled with how-to sex books and can "give a blow job as well as anybody." She doesn't have orgasms very often with her lovers—she waits until they leave and then gets herself off. When she invites a man to share her bed, she doesn't expect fireworks. She's truly surprised when she meets a man who is an attentive, imaginative lover, and gets a little uncomfortable when he focuses on giving her pleasure. "It's weird," she says, fidgeting nervously with a lock of hair. "I'm not sure what to do when a guy wants to make the night all about me. Usually I just flip him over and suck his cock—nobody can resist that for long." Kathleen doesn't feel she deserves being pampered in bed. Sex isn't exactly a chore, it's more like a sport. And she is sportsmanlike in her desire to play fair and avoid taking the home court advantage.

Kathleen is not alone among competent, busy career women who find the dating world competitive and unsatisfying. But even to the extent that they're right about some tough realities, that's no reason to give up on being self-nurturing and self-loving.

A Babe loves herself when nobody else is looking, and, of course, she loves herself when others are watching, too. But aren't you often a whole lot more sensually nurturing toward yourself when someone else is around to notice the result? You'd wear a lovely silky robe for a boyfriend, wouldn't you? But would you wear the same robe just because it feels good against your skin, just because you feel more feminine and sexual reading the Sunday paper all alone?

A Babe would!

A Babe is an erotically alive, sexy (degraded and lovin' it!) creature twenty-four/seven, just for herself. When she wants to connect sexually with a lover, she doesn't have to shift suddenly into an alien state of being, she only has to open up and show him the sensuality already bubbling within her.

Why do so many with-it and successful women like Kathleen have to learn how to become a Babe? Why isn't it something that really does come as naturally as breathing?

I Want to Feel Dirty—Not!

In many cultures, including our own, women are raised to believe that their genitals are repulsive and dirty. The numbers of women who have a hard time imagining why a partner would want to go down on them is a testament to this deeply inculcated message and to the cultural antipathy toward the way women look, smell, and taste "down there." How off-kilter is it that boys can have pissing contests, that men can line up at urinals wagging their little soldiers, but a woman wouldn't think of displaying the rosy petals of her vulva to another woman who wasn't a medical professional or a lover?

Not long ago, one of my close friends developed a medical condition that caused excess skin to grow over her clitoris. As a sexologist I was interested, and asked her if she would be comfortable showing the area to me. She couldn't bring herself to do so. She was too ashamed. I wanted to cry; as close as we are, this was off-limits.

Not only are we ashamed of our genitals, but we are also raised to perceive men as "experts" about our sexuality. We wait for a White Knight to "get us" excited, to "show us" how to come. If a woman with a partner mauls her own muff (!) the cultural perception is that there must be something awry in loveland. When a single gal oils her oyster, well, poor thing is just desperate and lonely.

BABE BOOSTER
Spend an afternoon walking around your house naked. Give yourself permission to touch yourself whenever and in whatever room the mood strikes.

These attitudes would be gut-bustingly funny if not so effective at keeping women down. The real pity is that we can sit around and dish with our girlfriends over the general ineptitude of men, their inability to grasp even the most rudimentary understanding of our emotional and cognitive processes, and still buy into the idea that these dolts should know better than we do what should make us squirm and gush and cry out in uncontrolled carnal delight.

I can think off-hand of at least half a dozen women clients who came to see me with sexual complaints ranging from lack of orgasm during intercourse (at least seventy percent of the women in the world don't climax without direct clit stimulation) to low libido (she didn't like hubby's six A.M. raging hard-on jammed in while she was half asleep). In every case the woman thought she had a problem because her man said so. His expert evidence? "My other girlfriends didn't mind," or, "My other girlfriends could come like that!" Thus, there must be something wrong with *you*!

The shame we feel about ourselves and our genitals, and our reluctance to stand up for our own knowledge about our sexuality—or to gain that knowledge in the first place—is part of a greater cultural conspiracy around what makes a woman desirable (or not) from head to toe, not just halfway in between. Why might you—a smart, sophisticated woman and a budding Babe, no less!—accept any of the self-defeating messages purveyed by our culture? From the most homespun wisdom borrowed from Mom, Dad, and Aunt Mary, to the glossily packaged conditioning stamped with Madison Avenue labels or 90210 zip codes, what sort of bull-dung are we making into bedrock?

Let's take a short detour to see how some fundamental and far-reaching cultural messages seep into our psyches and, it seems, our very cells.

The Bondage of Beauty and the Dilemma of Desire

Some culprits of conditioning are right under our noses, so familiar that we almost forget to give them sufficient credit for screwing us up. For instance, I don't think there is a woman living in America or any other modern society who in some way, at some time, hasn't felt in bondage to beauty. Good-looking women rely on their image as power, often unaware that the power is illusory, that their image is an identity so precarious it can dissolve in a flash through an illness, an accident, the ordinary course of aging, or the commonplace experience of gaining weight. On the opposite side of this distorted looking glass, a woman who is plain or out of shape might think about herself primarily in terms of what she lacks— beauty and the power it bestows—rather than what she possesses. Kathleen fits this profile precisely, even though her glib dismissal of men and her casual, utilitarian approach to sexuality valiantly disguise her pain.

A $33-billion-per-year cosmetics industry and a thriving plastic surgery empire pander to our anxiety about our looks and our perpetual attempts to enhance them. The reality TV show, *Extreme Makeovers*, fascinating as it is, magnifies the power of false image. Every makeover— whether subtle or extreme—is more than a stretch to be the best that we can be. It's an effort to clear another furlong in the potentially lethal beauty derby.

Oprah aired a show a while back exploring the connection between beauty, vanity, and self-esteem. Guests included a woman whose trademark suntanned golden skin was her greatest asset until a creeping melanoma destroyed half her face. Another guest invested in face-saving surgery for fear of losing her husband to a younger woman. She suffered nerve damage so severe that for the past seven years she has been bedridden due to crippling, unremitting pain. Her husband left her.

Deep down, each woman feared that she would not be "seen" if her outside wasn't alluring. Each feared that her inside could never be enough to warrant being desired.

The pity of our endless search for beauty is that beauty is neither love, nor passion, nor power. To feel deeply aroused and overtaken with our passion we need to be engaged wholly in the moment. This is impossible if we're paralyzed by fears about looks and rejection.

In one study, forty-one percent of 26,000 women admitted that feeling unhappy with their bodies was the primary reason for being unable to freely express their sexuality. Feeling reluctant to position themselves for intercourse in ways that are unflattering, some women avoid the placement they love most for fear of being exposed with breasts bouncing or belly flopping. The taut tummies and silicone-solid breasts of young models in adult videos are like flashing neon signs declaring to the average woman that if she doesn't look as slim and superb she shouldn't risk being seen.

Studies like this, as valuable as they are, miss the point that expressing sexuality is about more than coital positions—it's about expressing what we desire, think, and fantasize. By focusing only on the matter of body image, we may lose sight of the far deeper inhibitions that keep us from saying "see me" in less literal terms. See who I am, see how I need, see what I want from you, my lover. The focus on beauty, while cripplingly real, also keeps our attention off all the other layers of self that make our sexuality so very powerful and, yes, intimidating to men who would rather not see the desire they fear they cannot fulfill. How much easier is it for men to turn away from us than embrace our hugeness of spirit and yearning? But, Babe, just imagine how deeply we might actually hunger, how much boisterous desire could be coursing through us, if we weren't lured away from ourselves, distracted by bad feelings about the way we look instead.

The word "hunger" has many connotations. Beauty's pairing with slimness in today's world carries dismal undertones. Slimness implies (and actually demands) being controlled and disciplined. The lean woman is one who rigorously defies surrendering to her cravings. She trains herself to negate feeling desires to spare herself the torture of denying their fulfillment.

We live in a world where to be desired we must suffocate our own desires. It is no wonder that the incidence of disorders of desire among women whose livelihoods are beauty-based is even higher than among average women. So many shun the experience of real desire, as they are expected merely to project it. Having lived in Hollywood and worked there both as a therapist and within the entertainment industry, I have seen more than my share of this masquerade and, in my own way, and to my own detriment, lived with the pressures, too. When I was hosting the talk show on the Playboy Channel I was expected to look almost as good as the models, even though in my role as host I kept my clothes on! When my weight fluctuated during shooting you can be sure there were comments from the brass. When I left Hollywood and gave up the personal trainer, threw the diuretics into the toilet, started to eat real food and forgot to weigh myself every other day, I gained twenty-five pounds within a year. I felt at once relieved and terrified. I barely knew the person in the mirror, though I have grown more fond of her since then. And, not so strangely, I have never been so filled to bursting with desire of my own. The old me thinks I should get busy dropping down a few sizes. The new me cares about being healthy and toned but not about being thin. I still struggle some with this internal conflict despite my complete awareness of its insidious root.

What is the media saying about women when skinny stick figures are displayed as ideals on television? Aren't they whispering another dark and dirty secret—that women might as well just disappear? In a study of the effects of media on young women's self-esteem, researchers found that idealized images of rail-thin feminine beauty can send young female viewers—particularly those who place great importance on their appearance—into an immediate tailspin of anger and body dissatisfaction. If exposure to just a small number of commercials can have such an impact, we can only shudder to think what the cumulative effect of a lifetime of exposure can have.

Just for the record, let's review some alarming statistics. Eighty percent of women are dissatisfied with their bodies. Five to ten million adolescent girls and adult women struggle with eating disorders in the United States alone. Almost half of all American women are on a diet any day of the week. Does it ever end? There is a saying among forty-plus women that at a certain age a woman must choose whether to emphasize her face or her body. Scrupulously thin women look cadaverous as they age, but to retain the facial fullness of youth they need to grow a little broader around the middle. The same choice faces a Babe—you might have to decide whether you want to honor your face to the world or your body of pleasures. A Babe chooses sybaritic pleasures even if she doesn't quite match the slimness of the woman who remains ensconced in perfect self-denial. Being a Babe is about feeling desire and giving in to it. For a Babe, life is a feast.

But, even for Babes—whether we're size two or size twenty-two— when we live in a culture where women's bodies are repositories of shame, body love takes work. And that's why, contrary to what so many women believe, loving your body has nothing at all to do with what your body looks like. Even the most beautiful body is never perfect enough to be "worthy" of love because the shame heaped upon us as women threatens to disgrace and disfigure us all—if we let it.

IF!

Part of the balance we seek as Babes includes revering our bodies, despite all the cultural conditioning brought to bear upon us that makes a rather weighty project out of what should be as natural and easy as, well, a belly laugh! We can get there, but it means seeking body love from the inside out, not the outside in.

Celebrating the Body Electric

At least one group of women is demonstrating the importance of turning our backs on shame and venerating the beauty of *real* women. The creators of the Real Women Project (realwomenproject.com) in California have created a line of sculptures depicting ordinary women in exuberant celebration of life. Women of all body types, ranging in age from twenties to seventies, posed nude for the sculptures that aim to present an expansive view of true feminine beauty. Real Women is an exemplary, heartening project dedicated to self-respect and self-love. Yet, I believe we need to go even further—to extend our exhilaration in the body electric to pride in the body erotic.

Learning to value and trust your sexual body may take time, but, Babe, you have all the time in the world. You have your whole lifetime. I urge you to begin right now.

There is only one sure way to leap forward: giving in to pleasure, exploding with pleasure. Living inside your body and honoring what your body does, senses, and expresses, rather than living outside your body, gazing from a distance, judging, comparing, and competing. This is how you overcome.

ADORING YOUR WHATCHAMACALIT

We are surely more than body parts, but if there is one part that alone symbolizes our sense of ourselves as women, it is our *whatchamacalit*: our pussy, cunt, vagina, vulva, genitalia. We need to be grounded *there*, in love with ourselves *there*, connected *there*. We need to look at our pussies a lot, touch them a lot, make them real to ourselves a lot. We can keep from being abstract objects, things that are looked upon rather than felt from within by exposing ourselves (to ourselves) in a concrete, cunt-loving way.

BABE BOOSTER

While masturbating, purposely try to resist going to full-tilt. You'll quickly realize that suppressing arousal will just rev you up even more!

Many women consider this a difficult, even odious task. They fear that harsh voices will ring inside their heads: Don't touch. It's dirty. It's wet and sticky. Don't put your hands there. Don't stare at hers. Don't look at those nasty pictures.

Don't.

Those are tattered, decrepit messages and they need replacing! How about:

Babe! Let your vagina speak through wet, swollen pulsations and sing its own jubilant song!

When you're connected with your vulva, vagina—all the parts down there that have been shamed and concealed—you can link with the world in an essential way that draws you out of hiding and renews you. When you masturbate, you will be recreating the fundamental relationship with yourself. This is your core relationship, from which all other relationships spring. Sometimes you'll manage just a quick, "Hey, how ya doin' today, sweet pie," as you plug in and get off. And sometimes you'll commence a long, deep dialogue, a conversation with your inner goddess. The next exercise is that soulful dialogue, a ceremonial conversation, if you will.

Indulge in Sacred Ceremony

I'd like you to begin to think about the space where you yield to pleasure as sacred space and this exercise as a sacred ritual. During this exercise, self-touch is not meant to be an outlet for tension, a hurry-up-and-climax release, but a ceremony of indulgence in the delights of self-love.

This is a fairly long, elaborate ritual that unfolds in phases. You may want to divide it into two segments. Because women with varying levels of anatomical knowledge will be reading these words, I've written it with the more inexperienced woman in mind, adding definitions and descriptive maps to make sure that every reader is comfortable.

Use your breathing to help you remain anchored in your body, open to sensation, and free of tension. Remember the cleansing breaths you learned in Chapter 3? Use them now to ground you in your body: Inhale completely through your nose, exhale slowly through your mouth, lightly pursing your lips until all the air is gone, and envision tension drifting away on the warm wind of each exhale. A variation on the cleansing breath is the erotic breath: Inhale, imagining that you are drawing the sensations from the pelvis up through the center of your body, through your belly, chest, shoulders, and throat. Exhale in a forceful huff and— whoosh—let everything go all it once.

CEREMONY OF SELF-PLEASURE: PREPARATION

1. Set aside a two-hour period when you will be alone and un-interrupted. Turn off phones, computers, and television. Draw the blinds in the room you choose to use for this experience (bedroom or living room is usually best), and create a sensually compelling atmosphere with the use of scented candles, soft music, fluffy pillows to support your back on the bed or couch. Have something to drink on hand. You'll also want to have a mirror available

(preferably one that stands up by itself) and a bottle of massage oil. Finally, you'll need a good source of light, like a bedside lamp or desk lamp moved near the bed.

2. Turn on the light, lie back against the pillows with your knees up and thighs open, and position the mirror so that you can see your vulva (i.e. the full expanse of your external genital area). Spill a little massage oil onto your fingers and slide them gently over your genitals. Spread your outer labia with your fingers (this is the area covered with pubic hair), revealing your inner labia—the two stretches of protruding, more darkly hued skin—and spread the oil there. Add a bit more oil and begin to glide your fingers over your clitoris (the nub just below your pubic mound). At first, you'll actually be stroking the clitoral hood that protects this very sensitive bud. Then, gently pull back the hood to expose the tip of your clitoris. Spread the oil there as well.

DELVING INTO THE GARDEN

3. Think of your entire genital area as a bright flower, unlike any other flower in the universe. If you're familiar with Georgia O'Keefe's flower paintings, you'll see why they were considered so very controversial in her era—they are delicate vulva representations. There is great variation in women's intimate gardens: the size and shape of the inner and outer labia, the conformity or difference in their length and thickness, the tiny or large bud called the clitoral glans, the distance between the clitoris and the vaginal opening, the placement of the urethral opening (the tiny hole between the vagina and clit through which you pee).

4. Finger the entrance to your vagina lightly, and see whether you naturally react by pushing open or squeezing tight. Insert one finger gently as far as you can and try to squeeze around it with your pelvic muscles. Imagine that you are trying to stop the flow of urine while you're peeing. Watch as your muscles clamp around your finger. Squeeze as hard as you can. Release. Watch yourself squeeze again. These are the muscles of your pelvic floor known as your pubococcygeus muscles. You may have heard about doing exercises known as *Kegels* to strengthen these muscles, but more about that

later. Now run your fingers back a half an inch or so in the direction of your anus. Feel the smooth, tight tissue between the vaginal and anal opening. This is your perineum. The entire area you've been examining is erotically responsive to varieties of touch and pressure.

5. Without pulling back the clitoral hood, begin to stroke your clitoris again, this time in slow, light circles. Your clitoris actually just begins here. This is the glans, or head of the clitoris, analogous to the head of a man's penis. If you now press down a bit harder against the glans you'll feel erectile tissue beneath it. This firm bundle is called the clitoral shaft. Your clitoris is also composed of tissue that extends under the surface down the sides of your vulva, following the line of your inner labia. These are the clitoral *legs.* To help you picture this, imagine a wishbone. The entire clitoris is shaped like one. The glans is at the top, and the wishbone's arch is created by the clitoral legs. When you are aroused and the erectile tissue of the clitoris is engorged, the clitoral legs become highly responsive to firm stroking and pressure. Later on in this ritual, when you've reached a heightened state of excitement, try locating the legs by using two fingers to press firmly against your inner and outer labia until you feel the underlying stiffness all the way along their path. Notice where you're most receptive to stimulation.

> **BABE BOOSTER**
>
> *Turn your bedroom into a boudoir by adorning it in a way that makes your sexuality palpable.*

6. Let's get back to the gem that is at the center of your erotic universe, your clitoral glans, or less precisely but for ease of discussion, the pearl we're accustomed to simply calling the clitoris or clit. Switch off the lights and put the mirror aside for now. Sink into the pillows. Position yourself so that you can most comfortably reach your vulva with both hands. For the next few minutes, use the pads of one or two fingers to stroke your clitoris all over. Imagine that it is a clock. The top of the clit is twelve o'clock. The point farthest away from your belly is six o'clock. As you draw your fingers around the clock, stop at one o'clock, then two, than three, and so on, moving clockwise around the sides of your clit. Notice whether any of the points on the clock are particularly sensitive or especially

responsive. How strong are the tingles? If you are too sensitive for this kind of direct contact, move on quickly to the next step.

7. Now move your fingers slightly away from your clitoris so that you are "marking time" on the clock without actually touching your clit. You may be only a millimeter or two away, but you are stroking and placing pressure on the tissue that surrounds it, not your clitoris directly. Notice any new responses.

8. Your clitoris has been the center of attention for a while now, so let's explore the whole of your vulva. For the next five minutes or so, let your fingers linger over your genital area, using every style of touch you can think of: stroking, pinching, rubbing anywhere and everywhere, any way and every way. You needn't think about your movements deliberately, just enjoy collecting sensations and let your ministrations follow in response to the feelings they evoke.

9. Touch your vaginal opening, and notice whether you're beginning to get wet. If you are, use some of your own juices to create a slippery surface rather than relying on the massage oil as you continue to caress yourself. Once your fingers are awash with your own fresh nectar, lick them. It's good to know how you taste, and it's extraordinarily freeing to feel at ease tasting your own honey. This may be difficult to do if it is your first time, but be brave. Others have surely dipped their lips into this honey pot and loved the taste—now it's your turn to share their delight in you. And don't forget to use your breathing to help you pay visceral attention to your body.

10. Now, let's return to your sensitive clitoris. With so much stimulation it has by now grown swollen, engorged with the blood that fills the tiny pocket of erectile tissue and hardens your little jewel the way a man's penis stiffens. With one hand, continue stroking your clitoris in any way that's pleasurable. You're not yet seeking release, so if you find yourself getting close to a climax, back away for a while, and caress other areas of your vulva until the intensity recedes a few notches. You're going to try to build your arousal to a near peak, then let the level drop off a bit and build it again, climbing higher each time. If orgasms don't come easily to you, or if you've never had one, don't worry. This ritual is all about murmurs

of sensation, not climax. You want to loll in the nuances of touch. You don't get a better grade for coming.

11. With your free hand, begin to pet your upper body tenderly—your face, your neck, your shoulders, breasts, stomach. Stimulate your breasts almost as though you've never touched them before. Experiment with various strokes, squeezes, flicks, and pinches. You might discover a taste for very light, butterfly caresses applied to your nipples or for firm squeezes to your soft mounds. Notice whether breast stimulation seems to increase your arousal or cause distraction. If this is the first time you've ever tried playing with your breasts, don't be concerned if you feel a bit awkward or even annoyed by the sensation. In time, and with familiarity, you may find that breast or nipple play enhances your solo erotic experience tremendously.

12. As you continue to caress yourself, begin to conjure wisps of fantasy. Elaborate upon one of the stories you read earlier, or focus on a familiar favorite. If you go with something tried and true, add a new dimension this time, maybe encompassing a fresh insight gathered as you did the exercises in the previous chapter.

13. Don't rush; take your time. Continue to caress yourself as you evoke more vivid imagery. Let the scenes play themselves out like a mental movie. Change the particulars just a smidgen and run them all over again. Add a "character." Add two. Change their ages, their sexes. Switch to a new story line that places you in a role that's utterly foreign to your experience. Experiment with fantasies you don't even expect to enjoy, just for the sheer novelty. What do you have to lose?

14. As your arousal grows, you may get close to having an orgasm. Instead of giving in to your urge, slow your caresses or move away from your target in order to remain a while longer in this dimension of imagination.

15. There might be a point where you want to scream, "Alright, enough is enough!" You're riding to the top of the incline and you desire nothing more than to feel yourself crest. You've edged your way back from the same peak a time or two already, maybe more, now the combination of physical caresses and fantasies is drawing you

breathlessly to the precipice and you're longing to tumble over the edge. That's the moment to surrender all control and let yourself fly!

AFTERGLOW

The previous ritual was designed to help you learn more about the types of touch that give you the most pleasure, expanding your desire to seek a range of sensations, alone and with your partners. The more familiar you are with your own responses, the more adept you become in showing your partners the map to your pleasure zones.

You can show a lover how to give you ultimate pleasure by letting him explore your vagina, vulva, and clitoris at each point around the erotic clock—directly on and indirectly to the sides of your sweet pearl. As he caresses you, you can tell him where you are most sensitive, and what kinds of strokes produce the most intense response, using a simple one to five rating scale. Five means that whatever he's doing feels rapturous. One means you feel little sensation in that spot right now, but that could change.

BABE BOOSTER

Breathing can be a turn-on! Blood flows better when you're breathing, so you'll feel more intense pleasure if you relax and keep the air flowing.

You'll find that the same exercise can summon entirely different feelings when you start off at varying levels of arousal, as well as on different occasions. Our erotic tides shift moment to moment, day to day. Yet, some women are content to teach a lover one good trick and let him repeat it until she reaches terminal boredom. A Babe encourages mutual fascination with her infinite variations as part of the blissful sharing of erotic discovery and rediscovery.

I hope this ceremony will also:
- Give you permission to pleasure yourself freely, especially if you have been reluctant to do so in the past.
- Help you grow comfortable looking at and exploring your intimate folds, making it easier to do so in the future, whether alone or with a partner.
- Initiate you into the realm of fantasy by showing you the way to escape self-consciousness and make room for an adventuresome, daring approach to learning the language and imagery of your own erotic universe.

• Introduce the idea of peaking and pulling back from the brink of orgasm, which will intensify your pleasure when you do go over the edge as well as prolong your enjoyment of sensation and fantasy.

Squeeze to Please

Another way to intensify all the sensations in your pelvic region is to build stronger, tighter vaginal muscles. These will increase your sexual pleasure as well as your partner's, but you'll need to train.

You may have heard of pelvic muscle training as "doing your Kegels." This refers to specialized exercises named for gynecologist Arnold Kegel, who, in the 1940s, developed techniques to help women control incontinence by strengthening their pubococcygeus (PC) muscle. His methods also had a zippy little side effect—more powerful, easier to achieve orgasms and the ability to isolate particular areas of your pelvis, including the muscles around your clit or those around your G-spot, to heighten pleasure. The upshot here is that strength is pleasure—just like in those athletic shoe ads—although I doubt you'll be seeing PC marathoners "just doin' it" in Vogue anytime soon.

You can isolate your PC muscle by inserting a finger into your vagina and squeezing, just like you did earlier. Once you've marked the spot, begin exercising by inhaling and contracting your PC for three seconds, then exhale and release. Relaxing your muscles is just as important as squeezing them. You may even want to give a little extra outward push as you release. Inhale and squeeze. Exhale and release. Start off with ten repetitions and work up slowly to a hundred reps three times a day, increasing the amount of time you hold each squeeze to ten seconds (but you might want to take an extra breath or two when you get to that point). You might get a little sore at first, just like any exercise program. PC training needs to advance slowly. Back off a smidgen if you hurt. No gain with pain. Added variations range from imagining that you are siphoning water up, up, up into your vagina, contracting all the way to the top of the vaginal canal, to inserting progressively smaller dildos or vaginal "eggs" attached to incrementally heavier weights and holding them in place with your tough-gal PCs. You can also do the exercises very quickly, making speedy little squeeze and push flutters. Various resistance devices on the market work really well, too, such as The Kegel Exerciser.

This is spring-loaded—you squeeze down and it pushes back, enabling you to increase PC tone very quickly.

Ordinary Kegels can be done in varied positions: sitting, standing, straddling an imaginary horse, lying on your back with knees drawn back, on hands and knees, in your car, standing in line at the grocery. Look around you—if you're reading this in public someone in the vicinity is doing her Kegels right now! For added fun, you can even do your exercises while masturbating or having sex. Some women who practice the advanced techniques for years develop the kind of suction power attributed to certain legendary X-rated entertainers—the ones who can smoke cigarettes, suck up quarters, or shoot Ping-Pong balls across the room with their vaginas!

Super suction aside, perhaps the most important reason to keep up with your Kegels is to help you stay in touch with your vagina. Remember, knowing her, loving, being tuned in and grounded in your sexuality from the inside is how we overcome all the cultural yackety-yak that stands in the way of being the sexiest, most self-assured of Babes. Your vagina is you, Babe. Kegels are like deep breathing for your sexual self. Remember the sensory self-soothing I talked about in Chapter 3? Kegels are the epitome of sensory self-soothing and self-loving. When you are focusing on your vagina, you aren't driving yourself nutty with thoughts of pursuit distance—the old Sorry Six. Kegels are self-focusing in the most fundamental, ineluctable fashion ever!

G Marks the Spot

Because you had so much to do already, I didn't want to include finding and exploring your G-spot in the first self-pleasure exercise. Let's take a moment now to introduce you to this rather phenomenal zone, which can produce powerful, unpredictable sensations when properly stimulated.

First, though, let's talk about what I mean when I speak of the *G-spot*.

The "G" is for Ernest Grafenberg, the doc who in the forties and fifties published work indicating that this zone, when stimulated, could elicit waves of pleasure in women. The G-spot is not an actual spot or button—it is an area of spongy tissue surrounding your urethra that becomes highly sensitive when engorged with blood during sexual arousal. The area is behind the front wall of your vagina, about two inches inside on the tummy side. When you insert a finger, palm up, and then make a "come hither" gesture by crooking that finger, you are in the zone.

The area in question is also variously referred to as the urethral sponge, the paraurethral gland, Skene's glands, or urethral glands. However, regardless of the term used, we are speaking of the same organ, the female prostate, which is analogous to the male prostate. You can see why G-spot is so popular an appellation! Some women don't seem to have a G-spot at all in their twenties, that is, they don't react to stimulation of the prostate, and then in their forties, the spot miraculously appears, like some kind of cosmic booby prize awarded for having reached a certain age.

Researchers studying female ejaculation—the expulsion of fluid through the urethra that often accompanies prolonged pressure on the G-spot—have suggested using other popular terms such as G-area or G-crest because the term "spot" can be misleading. When a woman is aroused, her partner is likely to encounter a bundle of swollen, textured tissue on the front wall of the vagina, beneath which he feels something akin to a sack of tiny marbles. These are the glands that comprise the prostate. Although this is indeed what we call the G-spot, since the area is felt through the wall of the vagina, not on the wall itself, it might not be immediately perceived by a partner as marking the spot. Despite the confusion, G-spot has stuck and probably will remain the popular term of choice.

G-spot exploration is most easily done with a partner, because the area doesn't reveal itself until a woman's heightened sexual arousal creates vasocongestion—the drawing of blood and moisture to the area. When you are poker-hot and swollen, the G-spot can be felt as most distinct from surrounding areas. To feel the G-spot is to be better able to play with it—catching all the angles, putting pressure here or there or a little bit to the left or right. You need to be a trifle more the contortionist to manage this yourself, but it can be done, especially with the aid of toys developed precisely for this purpose.

To give your partner easiest access to your G-spot, begin by lying on your back, or leaning up against a group of pillows, legs open and knees slightly bent. If you're self-pleasuring, find a position that allows you to put your middle and index finger into your vagina with enough room to be able to move around some—on your knees with your seat resting on your calves, squatting, or even getting on all fours with one hand free to explore. You might also want to pick up a G-spot stimulator at an adult toy store or through any of the catalogues you'll find listed in the resource section of this book. A G-spot wand has a special curve that allows you to reach and place pressure upon the nooks and crannies of your vagina, including your G-spot. A particularly lovely and effective acrylic device is known as the *crystal wand*. Other gorgeous, artistic hand-blown glass versions of G-spot stimulators serve two functions— as coffee table art and as a love object.

THE JOYS OF G-SPOT PLAY

Before you begin G-spot play, keep in mind a couple of points. Begin when you are already highly aroused—don't go into it cold. Masturbate until you're near orgasm, or, if you're with a partner, make sure she or he takes the necessary time to get you toasty warm, highly engorged, and very, very wet. You want to feel desire coursing through you. You want to be silently screaming, "I can't wait!" for the next phase of discovery.

Pressure on the G-spot can elicit unexpected physical and emotional reactions, so no matter how hot you are, try not to rush. G-spot stimulation not only feels quite different from clitoral touch, but it can also facilitate profound emotional flooding. Remember that our bodies are the repositories of our memories, fears, and dreams. No part of your body holds more delicate feelings than your sexual zones. With G-spot pressure you might cry, even sob, especially if you have a G-spot-orgasm. In the course of G-spot play you might feel intensely vulnerable, so if you're experimenting for the first time with a partner, make sure you choose someone with whom you feel safe enough to be open and real, no matter what.

On the physical side, the G-spot can handle a lot of pressure, in fact, light stimulation is often imperceptible. Each square centimeter of the G-spot can respond rather differently to varieties of touch. Some women like certain areas stroked, pressed, and squeezed. Try alternating direct pressure on the G-spot with movement around the vaginal walls from side to side, or jiggling up and down with fingers curved, or in slow circles pressing into the vaginal wall at clock points. There's no need to limit your finger or wand action to the in and out that simulates intercourse.

Lots of lubricant or the use of tight latex gloves can feel wonderful because of their smoothness. The sensation elicited by each practice at various pleasure points can be different, too. Occasionally you might feel an intense burning, which can be oddly exciting or undesirable, or both, shifting from moment to moment. You may feel a strong urge to pee. This is normal, considering that pressure is being placed upon glands surrounding the urethra. You might want to get up to empty your bladder if you didn't do so before you began and then continue playing when you're confident that the feeling of wanting to urinate isn't an urgent message from your bladder. If you have that sensation again, you'll feel more secure pushing through it without using your PC muscles to clamp down and inhibit fluid release. Allow the sensations of pleasure to exhilarate you. Let yourself virtually explode into the feeling. As you continue to ride these sensations, you may very well feel the warm and powerful gush of fluid pulsing against your lover's hand. Surrender to this—moan, cry out without restraint. By diving into this pleasure you are quite likely to have an orgasm (what I call a G-gasm), perhaps along with an ejaculation of wet, wild wonderment. G-gasms can shake you to your roots, so be prepared to ride the tidal wave of both the physical ecstasy and the startling emotional aftermath.

Coming to Grips with Ejaculations

One of the most common questions I receive from women readers of my advice columns goes something like: "When I'm really excited (or, when I have an orgasm) fluid squirts out of me without warning. What is this?"

This is an ejaculation! Women can ejaculate with orgasm or extreme arousal, just like men do, especially if the right kind of pressure is placed on their G-spot. But the subject of ejaculation is shrouded in mystery and laden with controversy. I remember the very first time a "gusher" happened to me. I was with a new partner and I responded with alarm. "What did you do?" I cried out. I had a sense of being taken somewhere unsafe without having been consulted. All smiles, he said, "I had a feeling you could do that!" I'd never done it before, so I didn't know what made him so darn prescient, though once I relaxed into the whole experience I was thrilled with the outcome.

In order to help you let go of tension and enjoy whatever sensations come your way during sex play, it may relieve you to know that the liquid discharged from the urethra during extreme excitement is not urine. Researchers seeking to unlock the mystery of female ejaculation have found that the fluid is released in two ways. Stimulation of the female prostate produces an odorless, slightly milky fluid, generally in the range of three to five ccs. (Remember, the *prostate* is the anatomical name for the area we refer to as the G-spot.) The amount depends on the size of a woman's prostate: bigger gland, more fluid. Other studies have shown that women who gush amounts up to a full liter are emitting fluid from the bladder. However, this is also generally odorless and colorless, though lacking the diluted skim milk quality of the prostate's emission and containing twenty-five percent less urea and creatinine than is found in ordinary urine samples. Researchers are exploring the idea that the hormone aldosterone, secreted during sexual arousal, is responsible for chemical changes that de-urinize the liquid expelled from the bladder. You might ejaculate secretions that originate in the prostate or in the bladder or both simultaneously, because all of it mingles and rushes out through the urethra.

Both clitoral stimulation and G-spot stimulation can lead to expulsions of fluid, but by far the most common occurrence surrounds penetration with hands, toys, or a penis in the right position (often doggie-style) to offer prolonged stimulation to the G-spot.

Remember, though, that just as not all women have multiple orgasms, not all women have G-gasms, and not all women ejaculate. There is no reason why ejaculation should be a goal. It doesn't make for a better orgasm, it isn't a sign of greater sexual proficiency, it's simply part of what some women's bodies do naturally in celebration of the erotic. Far more important than trying to ejaculate is that you avoid trying not to ejaculate for fear that you will expel too much, upset your partner, or embarrass yourself. You are entitled to feel good about your body and all its fluids and products!

As further research is done, we'll learn more about the whys and hows of our body's ejaculatory pleasure potential. The crucial point to remember is that women are capable of excitement and arousal levels previously unknown to early sex researchers like Masters and Johnson. Sexology is a very young science and the "truth" about women's sexuality has been coming to light only slowly as the veil of silence and shame is lifted. Volumes of additional work need to be done. We need to make our voices heard and demand that science explain our actual experiences— rather than let the limitations of a relatively new science circumscribe the boundaries of experiences we allow ourselves to have.

The Last Taboo

Anal play is still laden with taboo, discomfort, and anxiety. Otherwise sexually uninhibited women still carry blocks to feeling pleasure in that "dirty" place. Understandable, being that we live in a butt-phobic culture. However, if you want to explore the full potential for pleasure your body has to offer, you don't want to ignore this highly sensitive area clustered with nerve endings hankering to fire!

To enjoy any anal stimulation, not just penetration, you need to relax your anus. Exercises using your anal muscles will help you learn to release tension in the area. Try clenching your butt muscles and holding for two seconds, then releasing for five seconds. Breathe out and envision a relaxed, willing anus.

You might begin stimulating yourself by touching around the outside during masturbation, or feel your rosebud in the shower as you lather up. When bathing, give your anus some extra attention. Stroke it lightly. Soap it, slide a finger in and tighten your outer sphincter around your finger so you can feel the difference between being relaxed and clenched. To penetrate further, you can use your finger or a small tapered butt plug with a flared base (for safety's sake, never use a toy without a flared base) and plenty of lubricant. You can even buy a vibrating butt plug, which can help relax the sphincter and feels fabulous—if you let it. You might even find it very exciting to insert a butt plug while caressing your clitoris dur- ing masturbation. Being comfortable with anal self-stimulation allows you to be more open to its pleasures with a partner.

Keep in mind that the tissue of the rectum is sensitive, requiring gentleness and lots and lots of lubricant even for finger-play. Thicker water-based lubes and silicone lubes are latex compatible and the best for anal sex with a partner. Remember, oils break down latex, so despite what you may have seen in the porn videos, forget the Crisco.

Anal sex with a partner can be highly erotic because penetration also rubs the G-spot from the opposite side, just as it rubs the prostate when men are penetrated anally. But going slow—slower than slow—is the secret to enjoying anal penetration. Relax. Lube up. Make sure your partner moves very, very slowly, one inch or so at a time as you adjust to accept him inside you. (Did I mention, go slow?) When you're ready, keep the thrusting slow, too. You need to be the one to set the pace for ramping up the activity to more vigorous levels.

Creating a Symphony of Pleasures

The beauty of knowing and loving your own vulva, vagina, anus, and all the pleasure points throughout your body is discovering how to play yourself like a bevy of instruments, mingling sounds and spectrums of sensation, moving to new rhythms, building to unexpected crescendos. You'll learn the kinds of stimulation that in combination are most gratifying. Many women have the most intense or multiple orgasms when clitoral, G-spot, anal, and breast stimulation are blended. And let's not forget the power of the PC squeeze! Others find too much going on at once to be so overstimulating that they feel less, not more.

There is so much to learn about pleasure. Alas, this book isn't big enough to tell everything! I hope I've incited your imagination and inspired you to continue your own journey into erotic self-discovery and fantasy cultivation. In the resource section, I promise you references brimming with advanced techniques, most of which you can do alone, with a partner, or even, if you are truly daring, with partners—plural.

Yes, I really said that!

Cavorting in Chaos and Complexity

In order to allow yourself to soar with sexual delight, you need to be unabashedly receptive to all your responses. Self-pleasuring to orgasm and ejaculation teaches you about your body's tricks and triumphs. Then, when you're with a partner, you have the confidence that comes from self-knowledge, plus the ability to show your lover what brings you excruciating pleasure, orgasm, and, if you're so inclined, ejaculation.

Every woman's body, every woman's responses to the slightest nuance of touch from one day to the next, is so personal that there is simply no one right way to turn on, build up, come to a peak, ride the peak, or dive into the mysterious spiral of liquid pleasure. To box yourself in or chide yourself over your uniqueness is to deny your sacredly female essence. A Babe revels in her femininity—she loves her spontaneity, her unpredictability, her cycles and tides so reminiscent of Nature herself.

Loving yourself and extolling your pleasure prepares you to take your sexuality into the world, expressed with authenticity, confidence, and an unbridled sense of adventure. At the same time, a Babe's sexuality is precious and meaningful; she bestows her gift upon others, but never foolishly tosses her treasures away.

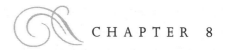

CHAPTER 8

Pure Exposure, Extreme Eroticism

Experiment creatively — within your comfort zone

S A SEX COLUMNIST, I often read other sex columns. When my
colleagues do something really well, they inspire me. When they
screw up, they show me mistakes to avoid. I recently came across
a staggering lapse of insight in a popular column. The advice seeker wrote
that her husband was on the verge of leaving her because after eight years
of marriage she couldn't get behind butt-fucking him with a strap-on
dildo. Here's the gist of the advice:

"Don't do anything you find morally repugnant, like watching kiddie
porn, but it's pretty lame to deny your hubby a kinda simple treat that
could save your marriage. You made it down the Hershey Highway a few
years ago with a finger and a prop, why be a party pooper now and refuse
to stick said prop in a harness and wear it? Try doing some research and
you'll see this can be safe, clean, and fun, and maybe you'll learn to like it
too. There's no need to strap one on every night—you can save it for
birthdays and holidays!"

The column goes on to spare no glib backdoor pun. Never mind the
inherent contradiction in the idea that a "simple treat" can save a dying
marriage. Beyond that slight of hand, I'm still trying to figure out how
turning the tables on a lifetime of sexual scripting without a pertinent,
penetrating fantasy life to support the shift could be as simple as tuning

in to a "Bewitched" rerun on the tube and, taking a cue from Samantha, asking the reader with the heart-wrenching question to fix her problem with a twitch of her nose. Can you hear her now: *Sure honey, twitch wiggle, I'll transform those tired old sunny side-up eggs into pancakes and sausages. Sure honey, twitch wiggle, would you like six-inches or eight? Not!*

Here we are casually talking strap-on dildos and butt-fucking, and aren't we oh so daring and open—but, tell me—how does the advice you just read address the trust, surrender, and forbidden pleasure the husband is dying to taste? How does eroticism happen with a partner who resentfully goes through the motions? Don't both of them deserve something more lustful than a wham, jam, thank you m'am?

Anal eroticism is very hot for many men because it massages the prostate gland—which makes it the male sensory equivalent of a good G-spot thumping. Plenty of women happily oblige with digits and toys, worn or handled. But, let's face it, strapping on a faux penis is not without out screaming gender-bending connotations, and for lots of gals the concept is too heavy to handle. Being the ravisher rather than the ravishee can light a fire in some women's eyes, and send others straight for the Xanax bottle. Think about it (as if you're not already!). Yes, if you are curious and eager and find the idea of buckling up to hump hubby hot, do it! Do it hard and love it, or at least love yourself for freely *wanting* to give it a try. But let's not ignore the host of meanings we bring to every sexual adventure. When we choose to experiment beyond the ordinary, the gargantuan questions that grab us aren't all vacuum-packed and sealed from messy emotions. They don't rest on clean, airless choices made because you love or you love not, either. Each unfamiliar sex act dredges up our enduring secret life, and right *there* in the crevice between thought and action, eroticism swells and overtakes us, or shrivels to nothing.

BABE BOOSTER

If you've always wanted to try wearing a strap-on dildo but are afraid you'll look silly and your partner will laugh, try blind folding him first. Let him get the feel *before he gets the picture!*

In an earlier chapter I talked about how erotic fantasies always conjure up the matter of power—who acts and who surrenders. Bringing fantasy to life incites *real* exchanges of power and control, real exposure of our hidden selves. Hot sex always asks what kind of exposure we can tolerate—how much, and for how long? The more exotic our activity, the more overexposed we get. Some folks try to shrug off sex games as just role-playing by sanitizing them with the "just" that leeches actions of their threat and melting heat—it's *just* a game. We're *just* playing pirate and maiden, prisoner and guard, inquisitor and suspect, daddy and little girl—all *just*, all light, fluffy, sterilized.

Sure, sometimes we can do role-play "lite," but mostly, what we do in those naked moments is slathered in meaning, vitalizing parts of our being, exposing ourselves in ways we find thrilling, terrifying, or trite. Nothing we do excitedly over and over feels unreal no matter how much whitewash we slosh on the action, because when it strikes us as *too* alien, we don't do it again.

Look at it like this: In life, we get to decide if we're gonna push the envelope or lick it. Babes are pushers, not lickers, but Babes also think about where they're sending their mail. In this chapter, we'll do some pushing, but we'll also keep an eye on the qualities that make every alternative direction so compelling, brash, and, yes, even devotional.

Exposing Yourself Like Never Before

Every topic in this chapter could be a book in itself, from bisexuality to S&M, gender bending, swinging, and polyamory. Each may seem like a completely different topic, but despite the diversity of subjects, when thrust into the vortex of the lived moment, these topics tell just one story—the tale of our erotic authenticity, revealed or as yet unexcavated. When we jiggle the swollen piggy banks of our erotic narratives, these shiny coins of complicit meaning spill out in a clatter at our feet.

This chapter, while falling short of an "everything you ever wanted to know" guide to exotic sexuality, will give you everything a Babe *needs* to know to support your curiosity, your yen to delve further—with lots of follow-up resources to help take you as far as you wish to go. I'll unveil the layers of meaning that give each alternative sexual style it's sizzle, and you'll be free to stretch and surrender your mind to the beckoning thrills. If you're single, I'll show you how to meander through these sacred gardens to find like-minded souls. If you're coupled, I'll show you how to invite your partner to join you in the celebration of your erotic spirit.

I'll begin with a topic that a lot of people might see as the most extreme or kinky of all—sadomasochism and its psychological counterpoint, dominance and submission. Why begin here? Because within the erotic landscape known by the shorthand of *bdsm* (referring to bondage and discipline, domination and submission, sadism and masochism) lays a power dynamic that, in less overt or conscious ways, *operates within our every intimate relationship.* When we tease apart the strands of enticement within this erotic world, we discover key themes that are embodied within other sexual elaborations as well. In the ultra-responsible approach to extreme thrills that has become the heartbeat of bdsm culture, we find maps to help navigate all our erotic journeys, even those which, on the surface, may seem to bear no resemblance to bdsm. For that reason, I'll take a little more time to flesh out this topic than I otherwise might. Even if you think you're not into any aspect of bdsm and were about to skip this section altogether in favor of one that makes the downy hairs at the nape of your neck stand on end, do read this anyway, as there's a lot to learn.

Power, Pain, and Pleasure

A few years ago, a survey by *Redbook* magazine reported that sixty-nine percent of women want to be controlled in bed. These days, it's a short hop from light force or a slap on the fanny to more extreme diversions. Movies like *Secretary*, for all its flaws, brought erotic domination and submission to mainstream audiences, becoming a *9½ Weeks* of the 0 generation (0 as in 2003-04-05). Yet this generation may actually exhibit more "O,"—as in *Story of,* than any before it. Never has a fascination with discipline and surrender, punishment and restraint, been so flaunted by the media, where glossy on-your-knees, boot-licking images in magazine ads share bindings with literary book reviews and elegant fashion spreads.

For a Babe, curiosity about the world of S&M is only natural. In fact, fantasies tinged with D&S (dominance and submission) or S&M are so commonplace among women that they're at risk of losing their *kink* cache. Uh oh! Power-exchange games are becoming the new normal—a scary thought for those who prefer to be different.

In day-to-day life, people have been playing with power in a subverted, unconscious, and nonconsensual manner since the beginning of human history. Even the most ordinary romantic relationships explode with power-struggle conflicts over who's right, who gets to control which aspect of the relationship, who can exert what kind of psychological punishment when their needs aren't met. Couples often play out their struggles aggressively over money and sexual issues. When it comes to sex, the partner who says no to nookie is always in charge. The one who craves more sex is stuck in the unenviable, submissive position of begging for blood from a stone, that is, from his or her passively commanding partner.

One of my clients, August, was slowly introduced to bdsm by a new partner when she hit her mid-thirties. She said she at first found it incomprehensible that one person would want to submit to another or that pain could intensify sex, yet her relationship history was actually grim with unconscious submission. There were the years of slavish devotion to unappreciative men that produced mind-blowing orgasms in the name of love. There was the time her ex-husband shouted in front of their entire tango class that he'd lost patience with her two left feet and left her standing on the dance floor all alone, rosy cheeked with embarrassment. There was the shocking moment when, on the drive home from class, August's tears prompted him to pull the car over on a dark side street and have his way with her on the hood of the car. And there were the hours spent primping and beautifying for a boyfriend who was more likely to point out a snag in her stocking than tell her she looked fabulous. August never called this adagio in self-abnegation "erotic humiliation" or recognized her endless attempts to please her men as exercises in submission gone awry.

Playing with ethical, *conscious* erotic power forced August to come to terms with the distorted power dynamic that had held her in its grip. Lovers' quarrels, love's tortures, and lovers' make-up sex had given August's life meaning. Only when she realized that these were perversions of healthy relationship patterns could she claim her own power during sex (and otherwise). Only when she began to use power consciously for pleasure did she discover that she didn't have to be a victim of power unstated, pain unwanted.

In contrast to the millions of secretly sadomasochistic relationships like those that littered August's past, conscious bdsm demands absolute consent between partners dedicated to mutual excitement and pleasure. Practitioners co-opt taboo in ritual episodes where power is the ultimate psychological sex toy and intense sensation is both a stunning aphrodisiac and an end in itself.

Bdsm is sometimes thought of as sexual theatre, complete with scenes, roles, players, and props. Certain themes are key to many bdsm experiences, and there would probably be thousands of story lines if one tried to tally them all. Let's turn to the themes now, for most of them will crop up again, even when we leave this topic. These themes include:

- Negotiation
- Consent
- Deliberate power exchange
- Challenge to sexual "norms"
- Exaggerated gender roles
- Expanded authenticity
- Pain into pleasure, pleasure into pain

Negotiation

When was the last time you talked about living out your fantasies, deciding who would do what to whom, *before* having sex for the first time with someone new? Well, in bdsm, detailed discussion plays such a crucial role that classes and workshops on negotiation are given at conferences all over the country. Couples negotiate about the range of their activities as a prelude to a scene—in bdsm parlance, the equivalent of a lovemaking session. Playing with power, bondage, and pain, or any combination of these—since not all people who love one aspect of bdsm love 'em all—means coming to agreements beforehand so that each partner is clear about the other's desires and limitations. Safewords are designated to make sure that no one gets more than he or she bargained for. Couples debrief afterwards, sharing what worked well and what didn't so that next time is even better. In ongoing relationships where bdsm is the hot blanket perpetually warming the bed, continued negotiations become part of the process of the relationship. As trust develops, one's darkest of dark desires bloom like night jasmine and become lighter for their exposure.

In "vanilla" relationships where sexual spice isn't bdsm oriented, artifacts of the bdsm world often slip in, for instance, light spanking, silk bondage scarves, or pretending one is completely in charge. These are all the accoutrements of fun sex, *de riguer* for hot monogamy, according to even the most conservative advisors. No wonder a study released by the Kinsey Institute in 2000 found that fifty-two percent of couples had tried bondage, compared to just ten percent in 1975. Such moments are rarely negotiated—they sneak into the bedroom by the side door. They may be an easy way to introduce an unsuspecting partner to your fantasy agenda without committing to anything serious, or they may be more than enough in and of themselves. If a couple finds these lighthearted adventures exciting enough to intensify, they'll need to start directly negotiating for safety and pleasure.

Consent

In real estate it's said that the key to success is location, location, location. In bdsm, it's consent, consent, consent. The slogan "safe, sane, and consensual" arose in the bdsm community to clearly delineate S&M from abuse or injury, D&S from coercion, and bondage from entrapment. The bdsm community as a whole takes pride in honoring and protecting personal boundaries. However, playing in this arena also demands a willingness to take responsibility for your communications to others. People do make unintended mistakes, especially when supplied with vague direction. Partners aren't mindreaders, and, as in any physically demanding sport, there are risks. This is a game for seasoned grown-ups who don't revel in blame or you-should-have-known responsibility shirking.

Deliberate Power Exchange

Power is the heart of bdsm. If wielding power is your rush, your lover's response to your control is your thrill and giving power away is the euphoria that keeps his endorphins pumping like a morphine drip. If relinquishing power is your high, then you want him to want you to surrender so badly he hardens at the very thought. Or maybe you switch, that is, sometimes you want to be in charge and sometimes you want your partner to *force* you to surrender.

Before we go further, let's cover some kinky lingo: A bottom is a bdsm practitioner who is the recipient of bondage, sensation-play, spanking, etc.

A bottom is not necessarily emotionally involved with the top or accepting of psychological control by him or her. If the bottom is more inclined toward erotic psychological surrender—following orders, wearing what she's told to wear, servicing the top sexually or otherwise—she might consider herself submissive. A top is the person who takes the active role in a physical scene but not necessarily emotional or mental control of the bottom. A dominant is more likely to exert psychological control, too. Some people can bottom to one person and be submissive to another, or submit to one and top another. This process of playing with power is known as power exchange. The conscious bottom or submissive is by definition a highly empowered being: One can only surrender power that one acknowledges in oneself.

Although terminology can be confusing, and different people imbue different terms with personalized layers of meaning, the very complexity and fluidity of these definitions underscores the role of power in bdsm. Even the adamantly nonsubmissive bottom gives up a great deal of control, and to whatever degree she surrenders or denies her surrender, there is still a confrontation with the aspects of herself that desire, fear, fight, or invite submission. Each scene becomes a physical manifestation of her inner drama, an erotic maze through which she chases her own shadows. And in the throes of a scene, the line between bottoming and submission will inevitably blur, or on the other side of the control tower, the line between topping and aggressive domination will smudge, and each participant will be forced to come to terms with that nerve-rattling ambiguity.

My client, Barbara, enjoyed light bottoming now and then—she loved to be tied up and sexually teased, she liked toys that hurt-so-good, that taunted her nerve endings, generating hours of exquisite torture, and she loved it when her partner yanked her back from the verge of coming, delaying her climax and taking her higher until she pushed Barbara's tolerances to their outer reaches and she burst into oscillating shock waves of sensation.

But "I'm *not* submissive," Barbara insisted.

Then Barbara met Tracy at a women's solstice festival, and Tracy, as it turned out, was quite the experienced top. Barbara grew to love, respect, and trust Tracy like nobody before, and she came face to face with the tiny demon she'd kept hidden from herself—her actual yearning to bob about in the sea of surrender without false superiority as her anchor to herself. Barbara had dreaded losing herself in a consuming love; erotic submission symbolized and, in actuality, played off of that fearsome loss, so she avoided the waterworld that held the greatest danger. Barbara's therapy emphasized honoring and trusting her strength and power, ironically emboldening her to give it up to Tracy for safekeeping from time to time. "I was so hell bent on protecting my power," Barbara whispered, "because I was so afraid it wasn't real. Now I know better."

Our lesson is this? Bdsm is a power-drenched universe. Role-play of any sort—including role-play that seems absent any bdsm trappings—is always at least splashed, and more often saturated, with power dynamics. And when we role-play, there's really no one to play but ourselves. We merely choose which of our hidden personas to enlarge or compress, which of our fears to accentuate or flee, and which costumes they'll don today.

CHALLENGES TO SEXUAL "NORMS," EXAGGERATED GENDER ROLES, EXPANDED AUTHENTICITY

S&M depictions in the movies and music videos are usually either over-glamorized or horror-laden, surreal director's visions, hard to distinguish from a supermodel convention or a psychopath's wet dream. When we wipe the slate clean of cinematic mythology, however, we find ourselves looking at a real life sexual alternative that is as individual for each practitioner as the mix of books on the shelves in their dens.

BABE BOOSTER

Men love control of the clicker, right? Wear a vibrating butt plug or clitoral massager on a date, and give your guy the remote control.

If you want to indulge in Victorian corsets, six-inch platform heels, or rubber suits, you can. If you want to collect bondage gear or play with ten-inch dildos and vibrating butt plugs the size of a pinky or a fist, it's cool. You can be high femme or ultra butch, regardless of your sex or degree of straightness, bi-ness or otherwiseness. The real feast is in the fact that sexuality is an acknowledged playground for the soul, a realm where relationships thrive on revelation and creativity. *Real*, even within the framework of fetish and fantasy, is where it's at. That's the part you don't see in the movies.

The lesson here is that you don't have to be into bdsm to extract meaning from the example it offers. No matter where your sexuality leads you, you can be all of who you are, expressed in any creative form you choose. Sexual freedom is your right.

Well, that's not exactly true—as a Babe, it's your obligation.

Pain into Pleasure, Pleasure into Pain

Love, when fiercely embodied, can torture with its dominating presence, torment with obsession, stun with its fragile beauty. Love hurts, not just when the relationship tears or shatters, but even amidst its cascades of joy.

Sexual pleasure, too, can peak and transmute into pain. We often seek shelter from an oncoming downpour of bliss before the agony of pleasure engulfs us. We resist crashing into a distant wall of pain when we don't trust that we will materialize on the other side in rapture.

The idea that pleasure can dissolve into pain stretches the imagination only slightly. The reverse is the greatest stumbling block some people encounter in trying to understand S&M. Pain giving way to pleasure. Isn't that...well...sick?

Consider this: Have you ever made love wildly, passionately, and felt sore the next day, maybe finding puzzling bruises or bites you couldn't explain because you didn't remember doing anything that hurt enough to cause marks? If so, you already know what it means to perceive erotic pain as pleasure, granted, on a light scale. When heavier sensation is applied, the body responds by surging with homemade chemicals, notably the endorphins, our bodies' natural opiates, which both diminish the intensity of felt pain and produce a rush, allowing ordinary consciousness to split away and hover in suspension—not unlike meditation or self-hypnosis.

Jeanne loves having pinchy little clips placed on her nipples and around her labia; she likes her boyfriend to use a soft leather whip on her inner thighs, bringing searing heat to her loins, and then penetrate her in the missionary position, pressing against those biting plastic clips, pushing the degree of pinch to the edge of tolerability. "I feel more inside. The sensation is so big, so hot, that I'm almost faint with it," she says. "During these scenes I can come just from intercourse, without any direct clitoral stimulation, because the contrast between the pain and pleasure amplifies the slightest sensation."

Is Jeanne weird? Not according to the latest scientific research. New brain studies have shown that pain centers and reward centers communicate—pain evokes activation of reward areas that previously were thought responsive only to such stimuli as drugs, food, and money. Maybe the "b" in bdsm really should stand for brain!

NOW WHAT?

Let's say that you've been intrigued by some aspect of bdsm for quite a while and you want to leap from imagination to action. What do you do? First of all, you'll want to check out the Afterplay resource section at the back of this book that lists books and Web sites chock full of further detailed information. Then, if you already have a partner, I'll suggest one approach. If you're single and looking, I'll suggest a way of safely meeting kindred spirits. You'll find this section toward the end of the chapter, because the advice contained there will apply to most of the other sexual alternatives we're about to explore.

EXERCISE Playtime!

Pretend that you're negotiating a bdsm scene. Based strictly on what you already know, what you've fantasized about in the past or read about in this book, what components would you include in your scene?

Would you want to top or bottom? Would your partner be male or female? Would you use bondage? Pain-play? Psychological domination or submission? Make a list—sort of like the ingredients in a recipe—of the features you're fairly sure you would include.

If you have a partner, would you feel comfortable sharing this list with him? If not, why not?

What aspect of you is buying into the rationale you just gave for keeping this exercise a secret? What do you still need to work on in yourself in order to let go of the idea that your partner's reactions have anything to do with your right to self-expression?

Woman/Woman Attraction

Given the extravagant palette of possibilities into which a Babe might dip the brush of her erotic life, woman-to-woman lovemaking is without question a primary color. One of the most common fantasies among heterosexual women is having sex with another woman. It's so persistent, in fact, that making love with other women is no longer outside the scope of the sexual norm, though for many women doing the unfamiliar is still tinged with discomfort. If one acts, the question arises: Does that strip away the precious "straight" identification that many women cling to in a world where bisexuality is trendy in some circles and disparaged in others? If you're a girl who likes boys, isn't it better to stay on your own side of the fence? As your mother has probably said dozens of times for dozens of reasons, why go looking for trouble?

MaryAnne is one woman who would snap back at mom by insisting that diversity in sexual experience is anything *but* trouble. She's engaged to a man she loves passionately, and, like millions of other couples, they plan on having a family and living happily ever—with one twist. MaryAnne doesn't expect to give up her additional relationships with women, and her fiancé accepts her exactly as she is, so long as schedule juggling permits. No, Mr. Generosity isn't gleefully rubbing his palms together in anticipation of his piece of the threesome pie—there isn't going to be much of that. MaryAnne protects her precious time with her girlfriends and likes to keep her partners all to herself. "These are satisfying emotional and physical relationships for me," says MaryAnne. "I can't compare men and women—they're so different. I love Jeff to death, but at least for now, if he couldn't accept my relationships with women, we'd have a real problem on our hands."

Is MaryAnne really a lesbian in denial?

Hardly.

Groundbreaking research into women's sexuality conducted by Lisa Diamond at the University of Utah tells us that much of what we believed to be true about sexual orientation and identity is just plain wrong.

BABE BOOSTER

Videotape your own lovemaking. This can be hot, but it also reveals how beautiful you look in the throes of ecstasy, or how you might hold back in the sack (often without even knowing it!).

Diamond's work blows the lid off the misconceptions revered as gospel not only by the average gal or guy on the street, but by psychologists and sexologists, too. Instead of falling into static, either/or categories, a woman's sexual preferences can be fluid and extremely variable throughout her life span. Can women who identify as lesbian have attractions to men and sex with men? Yes. Do women who identify as bisexual divide their relationships into neat, equal piles of men on one side and women on the other? No. Must everybody wear a label? No. Can "heterosexual" women have real love affairs with other women? Yes. If you enjoy sex with women does that automatically make you bisexual? No.

Sexual identity is chosen, not assigned, which is not to imply that one chooses to be lesbian or transgender. I am saying that no one but the individual has the right or capacity to classify or label her sexual identity. The myth that bisexuals are just confused gals unable to accept their "true" lesbian or hetero selves has been deconstructed, and so has the equally erroneous conception that "genuine" lesbian women don't feel a yen for men now and then. Thanks to research like Diamond's, science is starting to back up what many of us in the clinical trenches have known in our guts: The degree of a woman's sexual attraction to men or women can ebb and flow over time; the way we experience, identify, and label (or refuse to label) ourselves may change as our attractions shift in intensity.

Elise, whose last relationship of five years was with a woman, is now involved with a man. Her take is simply: "I love whom I love. Soul mates come in all genders. I don't want to put myself in a suffocating little box or pick a team to make other people happy, as if I were just betting on the Superbowl. If my current relationship ends someday, I don't know what sex my next lover will be. I don't even ask myself that question because I don't want to think so narrowly. I feel really lucky to be so open. Maybe that's my label—I can call myself *open* and be done with it."

Pamela has a different approach to same-sex attraction than either Elise or MaryAnn has. Her romances are always with males, and she enjoys an occasional sexual adventure with a woman who is not a close friend, nixing too much emotional intimacy with sex to "keep things from getting sticky." She prefers romping with a woman when her boyfriend participates, but not, Pamela insists, to pander to his fantasies. "There's something about Tim being there that makes the setup more erotic for me," she admits. "I like his hardness, the woman's softness, the interplay between all of us, together. I especially like him watching me…that's a huge turn on. With a woman alone, there's a missing piece—maybe it's a kind of male animal energy that boosts my sex drive and makes me hotter for both of them."

Pamela and her partner are careful about who they choose to join in their lovemaking. Just as in a bdsm scene, consensuality and negotiation are key. "We all talk about what we expect before we get naked," she says. "Tim and I learned in the beginning that if we just let things happen, somebody is bound to wind up confused or hurt, or one of us will get jealous or feel left out, so we have little signals now to let the other know we need their attention."

When we don't paint ourselves into little boxes and, instead, allow our erotic sense to engage, most of us are nonexclusive in our sexual attractions at least some of the time, and under some conditions. Why doesn't everyone act on these fluctuating waves of desire? There's the matter of opportunity—not everyone has a supportive relationship like Pamela or MaryAnn. But more often, it's the usual suspects—shame, fear, and political correctness—that get in the way of individual, fluid progressions, regardless of which way we lean. A Babe doesn't like to give her power away to such lifeless forces. On the other hand, a Babe won't leap into a ménage a trois because she feels pressured or because it's the cool thing to do. Rather, a Babe is ready to top the system, close in on her real yearnings, and stop to examine the physical and emotional manifestations of her attraction to women as well as men. Once she knows what she wants—that is, *if she wants*—she's willing to push the envelope of adventure and authenticity to its limits. When she's a great-grandma, she won't say: "I wonder what would have happened *if*.…"

Gender Bending

Gender bending has been part of lesbian culture for decades, but it has come out of the closet in bi and straight circles over the last ten or so years.

Women who play with other women, regardless of their self-affixed labels, often do so with a masculine edge. Nora finds that sex with a macho beat is her route to erotic meltdown.

"I love when a partner treats my strap-on like the real thing. I can even get off by having it sucked," Nora explains. "I like to force my partner's head down onto it hard sometimes. There's the psychological piece—I feel like I'm really being serviced, and then there's the physical thing—the bottom of the dildo pressing against my clit makes me come!"

Some women find Nora's attitude revolting, a shocking demonstration of what happens when the oppressed sex takes on the attitudes and behaviors of the oppressor. Others believe that there can be no oppression in a genuinely consensual act of pleasure, regardless of what that act symbolizes or might constitute in a different context. In fact, the subversive symbolism is part of the heat.

You don't have to be bi to find that playing with maleness and female-ness can be a thrill ride. The trappings of femininity can feel repressive to some women, caging them within a passive, socially ascribed role that is more easily escaped by wearing the psychic and material paraphernalia of maleness. Obvious accoutrements like a strap-on dildo add mightily to the illusion. The faux organ's essential utility aside, wearing one can catalyze gender alchemy, becoming the magic wand that Brianna needs to bring forth her "inner Brian." Suddenly, she moves differently, takes command differently, feels the power emerge from the casing of her femaleness.

Tina and her husband, Michael, are perfectly matched gender trip-pers. Wearing women's lingerie and makeup excites Michael; Tina gets off on guiding his dressing, then "ordering" him to serve her sexually. Their kink reflects an ultra-traditional sexual power pattern, where the "male" (Tina) retains the upper hand and the "female" (Michael) aims to please. In Michael and Tina's private universe, the story line alters abruptly toward the end of their sessions: Michael and Tina go at it the old-fashioned way with the equipment that nature gave them. When the spell of fantasy is broken, they snuggle like worn-out puppies, basking in the afterglow of sharing their erotic secrets.

Those who would judge Michael and Tina's play style might claim that acting out extreme power discrepancies is no more acceptable when the male oppressor takes on the role of oppressed than the other way 'round. I would argue that there is no oppression here. Michael and Tina are intensifying the magic in their relationship—the love, intimacy, and mutuality. Their ability to merge fantasy worlds and express a range of emotions blesses them, empowers them, and tempers the coils of their marriage.

When gender bending brings intrigue, fantasy, and aspects of our core self to center stage, we can dance to the irrepressible music of truth. When we clumsily go through the motions because we're afraid of saying no or risking loss—as in the story of the advice column reader at the outset of this chapter—we deny our truth, and the music dies.

A Babe does not deny her truth, but she does take a few chances in expanding its range. You might be surprised at how well suited you are for the as yet undreamed adventure.

EXERCISE Switch Places

Unveil your inner male in the middle of a date. Spend five minutes in the ladies room grounding yourself: Close your eyes, think about the kind of man you'd be on the inside, how you'd treat that "woman" you're with—the one who's waiting out there for you. Go back to "her" and play at being the guy for the rest of the night. Later, notice how differently you behaved (or not) and how you felt.

One Partner or Many?

Monogamy doesn't seem to work very well for the thirty to fifty percent of married people (depending on which statistics you believe) who cheat, or the fifty percent who divorce. Ethical alternatives to the one-sex-partner-till-death-do-us-part paradigm are mushrooming because not many sexually sophisticated people buy the idea that desire can be contained for decade upon decade without springing a leak. Rather than toss away perfectly good relationships for the kiss of a stranger, millions of couples are discovering swinging and polyamory, the two most widely practiced forms of consensual nonmonogamy within committed long-term relationships. A Babe may or may not pursue these options, but she should be aware of them. They prove that for at least some couples, you really can have your cake and eat it, too.

SWINGING

Nobody seems to know the true number of swingers—couples who have sex (but not deeply involved emotional relationships) with other couples—in America or the rest of the world. Estimates suggest around two percent of paired-up people, but because swinging, also known as "the Lifestyle" (as if there were only one!), is often entertained in secret, reliable figures are hard to come by.

Carrie and Alan have been swinging for three years. Once a month or so they attend a party at a swinger's paradise just outside of Seattle. Housed in a mammoth redwood lodge with retro-seventies décor, set against the backdrop of landscaped, parklike acreage, the club is one of approximately 500 in the United States. Not all of them are as vast or luxurious as Seattle's flagship venue. Some are redolent of sweaty, smoky discos, some seem more Elk's Club than sex club, and others have a homey and house-partyish quality, but they have in common a sexual *joie de vivre* spirited by couples dedicated to preserving the emotional exclusivity of their relationship while sprinkling it with sexual variety.

Carrie was introduced to swinging by a girlfriend who had been in "the Lifestyle" for many years. Alan was at first reluctant to consider the idea, not sure how he'd react to the sight of his wife with another man. But Alan and Carrie decided to attend a party simply as voyeurs, to gain a sense of the environment and socialize with others without feeling compelled to engage sexually. "We went twice, chatted with people, had dinner, danced, and then had sex with each other. Just hearing the sounds of people making love all around us was a huge turn on, and that was enough for a start," Carrie smiles. "On our third visit we met a couple that we liked, there was mutual attraction, and we plunged in. It was good to go slowly, because by the time we acted, we were primed and ready."

In the seventies, wife swapping was a male-centered phenomenon. Guys wanted to get laid, wives went along for the ride. Today, the lifestyle is almost matriarchal. Women drive the movement, warming to the sense of community and the opportunity to explore their fantasies. One professional woman I know tells of how she was the first to introduce vibrators to local swing gatherings in private homes during the early nineties. "All the men were getting off, but the women weren't so easily orgasmic in the group setting and needed a little boost." She brought her plug-in helper to a party and before long other women were doing the same. Among her friends, she was tagged the "Jean d'Arc of orgasm."

Swinging gives many gals their first shot at sex with women. In one of the few research studies of women in the lifestyle, a group of fifty women were interviewed; each had their first experience with a woman through swinging and prior to swinging had little to no fantasy orientation toward women. The researcher found that in the course of swinging, masturbation fantasies that included women rose from under five percent to sixty-one percent, and that every one of the women came to self-identify as bisexual.

Although I haven't logged much experience in the lifestyle, I am close to many people who have. I asked a number of them to tell me what they would want a Babe to know about swinging if she was interested in exploring with a partner. These are the words of wisdom I collected from people who represent a vast range of experience and swing styles:

- Negotiate beforehand what you'll do or not; discuss your fantasies and expectations and how you want to play with them.
- Have a safeword or safe signal so that if either of you is uncomfortable with something or someone, the action stops at the signal—no questions asked, no blame implied.
- Bone up on safe sex techniques; depend only on yourselves, nobody else. Not everyone is as responsible as they should be.
- Do every damn thing you want to do and not one thing you don't want to do!

However, avoiding what you don't want might be easier than acting on your desires. People often stop themselves from chasing down their dreams and settle for what comes their way. Afraid of living their fantasies, they go home disappointed. I find this to be a rather sad aspect of the lifestyle. If you want to deprive yourself of pleasure, why take the risks involved in alternative practices at all?

Once again, the core themes that arose in our discussion of bdsm appear in swinging and are taken just as seriously—negotiation, consent, sexual authenticity, and safewords.

POLYAMORY

Where swinging is mostly about recreational sex, polyamory is primarily about love and depth of relationships. Polyamory can be defined as the practice of building loving, intimate relationships with more than one person at a time, within an ethical, agreement-based context.

In my practice, I've worked with dozens of polyamorous couples and triads, I've taught workshops for therapists on working with poly clients, and, yes, I've briefly given the concept some personal attention. In the course of my richly varied experience, I've learned one thing for certain—polyamory is far from a panacea or cure-all for struggling monogamous relationships. Successful polyamory demands participants' emotional maturity and willingness to invest time and energy in processing relationships at a refined level of awareness. Polyamory is a complex topic, to which it is impossible to do justice in just a few pages, so consider this section a light introduction painted in broad brushstrokes—for pointillist detail, turn to the references in the Afterplay section of this book.

Amy and John have been married for ten years and throughout that time have explored various styles of polyamory. "The moment you step outside the strict boundaries of monogamy, structure is up for grabs," says Amy. "Polyamory is like a relationship salad bar—when you finish arranging all the ingredients, everybody's plate is going to look different."

John and Amy met when they were "poly singles," seeing more than one person, hoping to hook up with a primary partner who would not expect monogamy later. They now practice hierarchical poly—they are each other's primary partners, but both have a meaningful secondary relationship as well. "We also see other people on an occasional basis—we call these relationships 'tertiaries'. I know it sounds cold to label people in order of their importance, but all we're doing is using shorthand to acknowledge where our greatest commitments of time and energy lie."

Some poly relationships are group marriages, where three, four, or even more people share a home, incomes, and child rearing and may be sexually exclusive within the group. Some people see themselves as poly by nature, but don't always live an active poly life. They appreciate the idea that one partner will not satisfy all of their needs indefinitely and they like leaving a door open to the possibility of multiple relationships should the circumstances be just right. Still, they choose during long periods to focus on only one essential relationship. Other couples create a kind of hybrid between swinging and polyamory called swing-poly or social polyamory. These friendships involve more than recreational sex but are strictly negotiated to avoid being emotionally and romantically competitive with the primary relationship.

Of all the alternatives presented in this chapter, polyamory is probably the most difficult to discuss for the first time with a monogamous partner. Merely bringing up the issue of nonmonogamy changes the relationship paradigm, forcing the exploration of needs that are not being met and emotional secrets that have been kept.

Orchestrating a poly life demands that couples take a hard look at their need for grounding and their tolerance for change. To operate as though poly is solely about satisfying sexual or romantic appetites, rather than a context for living life as a whole, is to miss a crucial point—one that makes the matter of negotiation central.

Much like with bdsm, the foundation of polyamory is consent, which must be given at an explicit and detailed level. Amy and John spent many months negotiating their polyamorous agreements and continue to refine and update them as circumstances and the people in their lives change. "If any aspect of an arrangement is not working well for everyone, it isn't working, period," Amy insists. "Poly falls apart when people make agreements under pressure or lie to themselves about what they can handle. At first, poly sounds like an answer to all the pitfalls of monogamy—you get security plus variety, depth plus novelty. But issues often taken for granted in monogamy require tons of processing in poly, which means loads of work. John and I had to look at the big picture stuff, such as agreeing not to have sex with someone until the other has met and given thumbs up to our prospective lover, and the day in day out stuff, like deciding whether it's okay for either of us to have sex with another partner in our master bedroom, or agreeing how much money it's okay to spend on other people. Anybody who thinks polyamory is some kind of free-for-all doesn't get it. Polyamory is hard, and it demands a lot of you—so you'd better want it very badly."

Poly women are first up to debunk the myth that their love style is just another avenue by which men codify screwing around. They see poly as a means of counterbalancing cultural restrictions on women being in control of their own bodies and erotic destinies. "It's my way of refusing to put desire on a leash," says Amy.

Polyamory embraces the idea that we can feel emotions other than jealousy when our partner has another lover in his life; instead, we can feel delight in knowing that he is blessed by love. This is a simple concept, but we have few cultural reference points to support it. Consequently, polyamorous people get jealous, too, though they tend to view jealousy as less alarming than monogamous partners do.

Jealousy is always about fear. In monogamy, it is about fear of infidelity. In polyamory, it is about fear of the unknown and of change, fear of losing power or control in a relationship, fear of scarcity and of loss, fear of abandonment. Jealously may also be a sign that something quite real is out of kilter—something that should be known is hidden, a breakdown of communication has occurred, or important issues are dangling, unaddressed. Jealousy can be a signal, alerting couples to matters that need attention; it needn't be a siren warning of betrayal.

Like all of the other options touched upon in this chapter, polyamory is but one of many choices you can make in living out the promise of freedom and authenticity at the heart of being a Babe. Whether you choose to have one partner or several, rocky road sex or vanilla with swirls, a Babe knows that the limits she sets always reside inside the circle of what is yet possible and may some day come to be. Life is a daring adventure, and for a Babe it is an ever-evolving one.

Bringing Your Partner on Board

Introducing a current partner to your fantasy world for the first time can be the height of thrilling. It can also be fraught with complexities and laced with mistakes. Often, one partner is so gung-ho to involve her mate in her newfound (or long-held secret) pleasure that she overloads the partner with information or, worse, sudden demands, and even the partner who might have been intrigued if gently guided toward new horizons grows defensive. When too much is thrown at someone too soon, he may shut down. The watchword here is "easy," as in, "easy does it!"

The following four- or five-step process, tailored to your own special relationship, will help you open doors to spirited discussion while respectfully avoiding overwhelming your lover.

THE LEAD-IN
You'll want to introduce a new topic gently, whether it's spanking or swinging. The easiest method is a matter of bringing up someone else's

new experience and expressing your piqued interest. "You know my friend Melissa? Well, she told me about something that she and Paul did the other night that I thought was really hot. Want to hear about it?" Or, "I saw a woman on Montel who was married and had a female lover, too."

You are one comforting step removed from saying, "Honey, want to invite our neighbors over to have sex with us?" when you rent *Sex with Strangers* to view while nibbling on Friday night pizza, and then talk about the feelings the film evokes.

Viewing handpicked television shows, such as HBO's *Real Sex* and *Downloading Sex*, are superb icebreakers, too. These shows incorporate so many sexual variations that even outrageous quirks start to seem positively vanilla by comparison after a while. Just keeping up with the street interviews where couples are asked explicit sexual questions is a great way to open up to each other. If you were to do nothing more than answer all the questions asked by the shows' producers, no topic would remain a sacred cow for long.

THE SHARE

Soon after you introduce a topic in a generalized way, you'll need to cough up the explicit images your imagination holds. Here's where being a bold and authentic Babe pays off. What self-respecting Babe is afraid to tell the truth about her fantasy life? Sharing your inner world is the first step to bridging the gap between what you think about and what you sincerely want to do. Your partner's fantasies may not mirror yours exactly, and he might not have yet dared go exactly where yours take you, but that doesn't mean he won't be inspired by the new and different. Of course there's the risk he'll run for the hills, but you can work around that, too. (Have strong bolts installed on your doors and wear the only key on a chain around your neck!)

THE REACTION

If your honey jumps at his chance to don a black leather mask, break into your house, and act out a rape scene with you, then you only have to consider the parameters of negotiation. How do you do this safely? What will you wear? Success is ultimately in the details, and to keep you on track I advise you make use of the references I've provided at the end of the book. (Of course, if your sweetie jumps *out* the window after hearing the plotline of one of your tales, you have a different situation on your hands!) When a scene goes wrong, it can go very wrong; that's why you need to educate yourselves before advancing too far. Reading books or renting films on how to explore new sexual horizons safely can be a hot exercise when shared, too. Don't skip over the excitement of learning together just because you want to get to "the good stuff." *It's all good stuff.*

But, seriously, what do you do if your honey's reaction isn't immediately positive? Give up?

No way. Not if you're a bold and bodacious Babe!

THE REWRITE

If the sexual script you revealed didn't immediately steam up your darling's glasses, give the subject a rest for a few days. Then approach again. Only this time, ask about his sexual secrets. After all, you've shown him yours, now it's his turn. If you genuinely like his ideas, let him know how *much* you get off on them and begin to loosen the restrictions on your sex life by being receptive to playing with his tastes. I know, I know, you're not thrilled about catering to his needs first. You want some attention to yours, especially now that you've finally drummed up the courage to reveal them. It's only fair.

There's danger, though, in becoming withholding because your fantasy was spurned. The unvarnished truth is that the more inclined you are to embrace his fantasies, the more likely he will be to loosen up about yours in time. Once a few walls have crumbled, he'll be more daring. It may take time—he may not be as Babe-brave as you—but a Babe is patient when she knows what she wants.

THE SEDUCTION

Sometimes you have to show 'em, not tell 'em. All the talking in the world isn't going to light a guy's fire if he's put off by the unfamiliar simply because it's unfamiliar. For example, if you usually go along with whatever your lover wants and now hanker to turn the tables, merely discussing power exchange might lack the verve and vixenish assertion he needs to shrug off his usual role. You're going to have to give him a sample. Show up at the door dressed like a dominatrix and order him to strip; tell him to lie down on the bed and be a good boy while you ravish him with your mouth, or make him do your bidding. Sure, he might laugh, and nervousness will kick in, but if you act like the hellcat in latex you're dressed to be (and don't get a giggle fit yourself!) he'll probably succumb to your control in spite of himself. Afterward, you can talk about how he felt submitting to you, and whether he'd be willing to make such a scene a regular part of your repertoire.

On the other hand, if you want him to be more aggressive—and because he's such a nice, sensitive guy, he bristles at the very idea of any Neanderthal displays—you give "topping from the bottom" a go.

BABE BOOSTER

Your voice is a hypnotic instrument. Use it to lull, cajole, and seduce. Touch your lover with your voice in soft, slow, low caresses.

Dress the part of slinky submissive and treat him with very subtle deference, the kind that's easily mistaken for a "let me pamper you tonight, baby" approach. Maneuver yourself so that his body is at some point pressed forcefully against yours and say, "I love it when you hold me down like that...don't let me move...I want to feel helpless...tell me I'm not allowed to even twitch a muscle, or else!" And later, "slap my bottom, hard...oh, honey, that really sends tingles like electricity straight to my pussy! Can you do it harder? That's great, yes, yes, again!" And later still, "I love it when you tell me how to please you, it makes it so much easier for me to give you what you want. Please tell me exactly what you want me to do to you, now. I want to hear the words."

You get the picture? Later you can talk about how he felt hearing you egg him on like that—how he felt aggressing upon you—and you can describe effusively how his dominating style affected you.

The unknown can be scary, even for a guy who pretends to know everything! When he's already hot and heaving, though, if he can be seduced and inspired to taste the forbidden, he'll usually find it far sweeter than he anticipated. The trick here is your own ability to get past reluctance to ask for what you want, or in some instances, to out and out take it.

Finding a Mate for Fantasy Play or Long-Term Love in the Kinky Kingdom

If you're single and you'd like to connect with someone who has a taste for the exotic erotic, whether for adventure or in the hopes of finding a long-term partner who shares your curiosities, you have interesting options open to you.

You're probably already doing the single-mingle, meeting candidates in the usual venues: clubs, work, through friends, maybe via Internet or newspaper personals, speed-dating, or travel. But chances are, you aren't bringing up your sexual tastes or curiosities at the outset of your acquaintanceships, even if you hook up for sex now and then. My question to you is: Why not?

Here's where we separate truly bold, authentic Babes from little lambs in Babe-imitation crimson bustiers.

You will never have a better opportunity to set the stage for a new relationship than at the outset. You have nothing to lose but your inhibitions.

If you want to go straight to the heart of the matter, you can make a point of meeting people in environments already conducive to exploring sexual alternatives. For locating these windows on the world, the Internet is your friend. When I began writing this section, I already knew key sites for both personal dating and links to social groups in various cities, but just for fun I plugged the phrase "how to meet kinky people" into the Google.com search engine. Lo and behold, I was immediately greeted with page after page of links—many new and thriving—that offered opportunities for meeting online as well as in person in cities across the United States and abroad. Then, for a little more fun, I plugged in "meet kinky people" plus the name of a city that might be considered more bible belt than studded belt, more folksy than free-spirited. I went through this routine for about eight randomly selected metropolitan areas, none of which were in California, New York, or Washington (hubs of exotic erotic activity), and again, *voilà*, I found a surprising variety of options for meeting the needs of anyone seeking spice with their sex. In the Afterplay section, I have listed links to some of the largest sites, but for now, let's talk about the plusses of using the Internet as your key to the kinky kingdom.

CONTACT WITHOUT COMMITMENT

If you're curious about venues for meeting others, cruising the Internet is like taking a long drive in a limousine with darkly tinted windows—you can see the world in protected comfort, but the world can't see you. Whether you catch a glimpse of newsletters detailing happenings in your town, stumble across online journals or *blogs* written by members of local alternative sexual communities, or freely browse dating sites, you can get the flavor of the scene before venturing forth in the flesh.

You'll notice that many cities have casual gatherings for people interested in bdsm. Called munches, these are usually held in coffee shops or restaurants, where you can meet without any pressure to hook up. When you're ready to step out of hiding, these chaste social opportunities are red carpet opportunities for exploring your city's kinky byways. Eventually you may want to attend public "play" venues. You can socialize and be a voyeur to the action without participating, but it's often more comforting to attend these events with people you've met through other means rather than go alone. The same holds true for poly social groups as well as swing parties. Even though many swing clubs welcome a limited number of unescorted women, for the uninitiated, going solo is usually too anxiety producing, especially if you aren't sure you want to launch into any action.

INTERNET COURTING SITES

Just like your average dating site, alternative personals offer photo displays and profiles, but unlike the vanilla variety, these can range from basic descriptions of one's dream guy or gal to the most explicit details of sexual experience. Fill-in forms denote level of interest in and experience with every imaginable style of sexual and S&M play. Going this route is like writing your tastes in neon—it's fine for your prospective dates, as the info will give you plenty to go on, but probably not wise to take that route yourself. There's the matter of too much information, especially if you post a photo online. Does your coworker or brother-in-law need this much detail? (You never know who browses these sites just out of voyeuristic curiosity!) Save the play-by-plays and the comparison of elaborate forms for later in the process with someone who appears to be a good candidate for body bonding.

In alternative matchmaking, as with any other kind, safety is a primary factor to consider, not because there are more prospective serial killers in this bunch—there are not—but simply because when erotic tastes are out in the open, some sleazeballs will try to capitalize on the free exchange of sexy chat, even if it's behind their wives' backs, with no intention of pursuing a real-time relationship. However, Internet introductions allow you time to get to know a guy (or gal) online. You have a chance to see how he operates, and usually, the same telltale signs of a jerk in real life point to one in the cyber world. Only if everything checks out do you progress to talking on the phone, and then finally to meeting face to face.

For women on the Net, there is protection afforded by common cyber-dating etiquette. Within cyber communities, women are advised to be especially cautious about revealing personal information early on and men to be more forthcoming with facts that can be checked out. Sexist rules? Maybe. I've heard some men complain about the unfairness, and usually they're nice guys who feel vulnerable, too. But sometimes, they're the same guys who have something to hide—at best, they're married and sneaking around the cyber backdoor; at worst, they really are predatory, scary dudes, and you want to steer clear of them in either case.

The rules often relax a bit if you're a woman seeking another woman. Alternative personals give you this option, too, and sometimes it's a far better choice than trying to seduce one of your friends, especially if it's your first bisexual adventure. Each woman needs to decide how much information she's comfortable revealing, and respect one another's boundaries. Men sometimes pose as women, so until you have a phone conversation and a real meeting, it's best to be less disclosing than you are accustomed to being with other women. Couples also place personals looking for a third for frolicking. If you decide to pursue a couple, the standard cautions about male/female engagement apply here as well. Whether your dates are with men or women or both, always meet for the first time in public, well-trafficked places. Take your own car on the first few dates and always arrive and leave separately. If you decide to get cozy with someone you meet online, arrange a "safe call" with a friend who knows all your date's vitals, and make sure your date knows you have made this arrangement. A safe call obligates you to be at a specified place at a certain time so that your friend can phone and confirm that you are okay.

Yes, it musses with the spontaneity, but a Babe considers safety first so that she needn't be sorry later. A Babe takes her sexual freedoms seriously enough to approach wisely.

In fact, the cautions that apply to online courtship could apply to any meeting of new partners. Although liars and cheaters are known to ply their craft on the Internet, they also pop up at nightclubs, parties, and even the Starbucks down the street. Sometimes even well-meaning friends can be fooled and hook you up with a loser. The most insincere, predatory man I ever dated was introduced to me by a trusted friend! Goes to show that regardless of where or how you meet someone, dating is never risk-free. On the other hand, I met a man on the Internet while I was researching an article about cyber-dating who proved to be all he advertised and more, and we dated seriously for more than a year. Personally, I find the Internet to be a few degrees safer than being out in the streets because we are naturally more guarded—we expect potential partners to prove themselves before we leap into martinis, let alone bed!

In the alternative personals world, some folks are looking for relationships, some for uncomplicated sex or bdsm-style play, some for ongoing, nonmonogamous partnerships. Make sure you know what you're looking for, and choose wisely. Just for the record, there's only one fantasy that has no place in a Babe's universe—a man who says he wants no-strings sex, or says he's polyamorous, and you imagine, "When he meets the right woman, he will change." Actually, I'd call that a delusion, not a fantasy. If you expect a miraculous turnabout, you'll be setting yourself up for some deep down, serious hurt. One rule to tuck under your pillow: A Babe does not enter into new relationships thinking she can change people or seduce them into being someone other than who they really are!

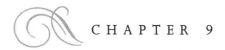

CHAPTER 9

Babes in Action

*Follow the foolproof Babe rules of your sexual
fairy godmother*

I F I HAD TO STRIP the essence of being a Babe down to one sentence
it would be this:

A Babe feels fully entitled to love wisely, to speak up, to feel, to sex.

It's a short, simple sentence, but it is power packed with significance.
It means that it's up to you to actively, passionately seek expression of
your eroticism and sexual curiosity. Dismiss externally imposed limits.
Accept no one's judgment, and refuse to justify your choices to anyone.

In the last chapter you were introduced to just some of the possibilities available to a Babe who seeks both adventure and deep meaning.

However, the world poses both pleasures and dangers for the brave,
newborn Babe. Many sexual explorers presented with such an expansive
menu are overwhelmed by the sheer bounty available to them and often
dismayed by the anxieties each option provokes. How do you decide
what will work for you? How far beyond the safe confines of your private
fantasy life or your steady relationship's customs can you venture? How
do you avoid sliding into old traps, into patterns of fusing and giving
yourself away, only in elaborately camouflaged forms?

Like the aerial artiste, how can you be sure that when you grasp hold
of the trapeze and swing boldly out into space, there will be a net
beneath you? So many questions. For some women, too many. Fear of
error engulfs. Those all-inhibiting social messages and, worse, that nasty

internal finger pointing, rise up again. Just when you most want to stretch out to meet the bar, someone down on the ground cries out in warning. You resign yourself—real adventure is too bewildering, maybe too pricey.

Remember! You have options: In love affairs you can have depth or you can have intensity.

Pick one.

In your affair with life, you can have exhilaration or erotic stagnation.

Pick one.

A Babe lives daringly. A Babe lives wisely. These are not contradictions.

Daring Do's Your Mother Never Taught You

Developing discrimination, resilience, and ultimately an inner wisdom will take time and practice. That's why, as a novice adventuress, you need a sane and simple plan to help steer you through the labyrinth of uncertainties. You need a set of universal Babe rules for living large and juicy. And that's exactly what I'm about to give you: The rules your mother never taught you.

Even if your mom knew these rules, she probably wouldn't have shared them with you. Moms insulate their daughters from the monsters that live in the dark corners of their own sexual psyches. Moms are the voices on the ground, halting you as you extend your arm toward the trapeze. Her warnings are meant to spare you from getting your heart smacked around, getting your body bruised. These and other loathsome prospects clutter the imaginations of loving mothers, whose basic urge is nesting and protecting. You can't blame them for trying to keep you safe, but in their efforts they often forget that you won't grow strong unless you are tested, stressed, tested, stressed, again and again.

Here are the rules for sexually adventurous Babes that will both challenge you and make you stronger. Some of these rules will revisit messages you've heard earlier in this book. That's because I wrote these rules to stand alone. If this is the only chapter you choose to re-read when you need a gigantic Babe Booster, it will be complete. Let this underscore previous messages, flesh out topics that have been only touched upon before, and add new, empowering ideas.

1. Surrender to Your Eroticism

Your seventh sense is always turned on. Live it. Breathe it. Walk it. Wear sex like a string of pearls around your hips. Hell, wear a string of pearls around your hips! Wear a lace thong to have tea with your grandmother. Wear fuck-me pumps to a business meeting. No one but you will know how or why you exude such palpable sensuality.

I saw a rather apropos commercial on television just the other day. The scene opens as a dashing African-American man in his forties—a totem of ageless masculinity and virility—struts down an office corridor collecting the admiring glances of coworkers. Every few seconds one of them asks a significant question: Have you been promoted? Lost weight? New suit? Won the lottery? The man's answer is a slight shake of his handsomely sculpted head, eyes gleaming, a barely discernible grin nipping at the corners of his mouth. After running a gauntlet of questions, he reaches his private office and settles down behind his desk. The name of the advertised product now flashes triumphantly across the screen: VIAGRA.

Our hero owes his newly engaging carriage to a pharmaceutical, and the world has taken notice. Everyone can see the transformation, they just don't know what caused it.

As an amusement, the commercial walks softly, but it carries an even bigger stick than the one I couldn't help imagin-

> **BABE BOOSTER**
> *Be careful what you wish for! Asserting your desire means being ready and responsible to handle what you've got coming....*

ing in tumescent levitation. The ad reminds us that, male or female, when we focus our attention on sexual pleasure, our aura shimmers with power and pride, and onlookers respond. That invisible outpouring of energy can trump a Wonderbra or a midriff tank any day of the week. Steeped in the hip swish, the wet wiggle, the wild will of our eroticism, we could even wear burlap sacks and librarian hair and there would be no overlooking our seductive glow.

In a reported interview with Eve Ensler, the creator of the hit stage play *The Vagina Monologues*, Ensler talks about how working on the play changed the way she relates to her own sexuality, her own vagina. Ensler uses the term vagina broadly, much as Inga Muscio uses cunt as the anatomical jewel that encompasses the totality of her sexual vitality.

Ensler talks about how a consciousness of her vagina means that when she walks into a room, all of her enters. When she writes, she is completely engaged. When she is having sex, she's whole, not dissociated. She believes that when a woman connects with her vagina, she connects with her desire, and when she connects with her desire she comes into her ambition, and she can give herself, without giving up her will or needs. The woman who desires, says Ensler, is able to ask for what she wants and take what she wants, something women are not brought up to do. Ensler admits that when she first became conscious of her vagina, she was scared to feel so much desire all the time and part of her wanted to shut it down. To feel desire is to feel *definite*, she says. And that can be terrifying.

Ensler is right. Being keyed into what I call eroticism and she calls vagina and Muscio calls cunt can be excruciating. But once you have connected to yourself in so powerful a way, once you have discovered the secret that the world tries to keep hidden, turning away is even more frightening. Waking up to your eroticism may leave you quaking at first, but, in time, feeling so alive, so definite, is a feeling of being home.

2. Keep on Fantasizing and Fantasizing and Fantasizing

Stain your brain with fantasy. Let cadmium and ochre and blood red images coat your world. Keep your imagination primed by reading erotic stories and poetry. Search out erotica on the Internet and in literature, photography, and art. Be chilled, aroused, sated. Don't let excuses and ordinary demands interfere. Inter-*fear?* Avoidance of fantasy is a manifestation of fear of pleasure, fear of power, a reminder of the tattered cultural lessons that have no place in a Babe's life.

The previous chapter was devoted entirely to living out some of the fantasies you may have only begun to behold or understand. Making the switch from enclosing a fantasy in the bell jar of your psyche to giving it flesh and form is like going to boot camp for boldness. If you have a partner, you know that living out a fantasy means sharing your story with him, and, as I mentioned earlier, that can be rattling.

One of the fantasies women often harbor is making love with their partner and another man. When the typical reader of one of my columns brings up the issue, she has already made the suggestion and her partner has accused her of demanding his right testicle in a bowl. (Naturally, he thinks his fantasy of enjoying her with another woman is perfectly dandy.) His reaction only reinforces her original hesitation to reveal herself. She regrets ever raising the issue, and now her precious fantasy, perhaps shared in the boundless blush of closeness following lovemaking, seems tainted. Her story has become all about him—his emotions, his perceptions, his need for her to enter his paranoid world, his trampling upon her rarefied dreamscape. Perhaps, she thinks, she should hold her other fantasies in reserve, too.

In my response to her letter, I always urge her to protect her lusty visions from his homoerotic anxiety—the standard-issue fear of touching and being touched by another man. Perhaps in time he'll find that it's safe to play with the right person, but even if he balks indefinitely, he can't be allowed to spoil her fantasy. Yet, continuing to invite him into her fantasy world is crucial to their intimacy.

Her guy can grumble, but a Babe remains faithful to herself, to the content of her dreams and to the rough edges of her desires. This is how her balance is tested. A Babe's sexual fantasies are like her political ideals or her spiritual beliefs. She doesn't give them up because her partner scoffs. She might decide not to act on a particular fantasy if her relationship is monogamous and her lover is opposed in honor of her *reciprocal* agreement with him. She would expect the same consideration were their roles reversed. But her appreciation of her desires and her pride in them must remain unsullied.

3. Rip up Your Labels

In her one-woman stand-up show *I'm the One*, comedienne Margaret Cho does a bit about performing on a lesbian cruise ship ("Eight hundred lesbians—so much DRAMA!"). She says: "I had sex with this woman on the ship and I went through this whole thing: Am I gay? Am I straight? And I realized—I'm just *slutty!*"

I wish she'd said, "I'm just a BABE!" But, hey, she made the point.

Labels belong in the waistband of your jeans, not applied to your sexuality. Labels have nothing to do with what makes you squirm inside those jeans, or who gets to rip them off. Authentic sexuality is about pleasure and connection, and pleasures have names—like Ted and Mary—not labels.

I often receive questions that run along the lines of "My boyfriend likes to slap my ass during foreplay. Is this S&M?" or, "My boyfriend likes me to insert my finger in his ass. Is he really gay?"

Labels are annoying because they imply limitation and, depending on the values you ascribe to them, they confer coolness or lack of it. For example, in circles where it is stylish to be bisexual, that label is applied with the precision of using a spray gun to polish toenails. In circles where it's common for young women to make out with other girls at parties for the voyeuristic pleasure of boys, the *bi* label is rejected for all the wrong reasons, as it suggests you're getting it on with gals because doing women is *your* thing, rather than just for the benefit of *his* throbbing thing. In such cliques, that's a no-no because male gratification is the only point.

Ripping up labels is not done to make others, including horny boys, parents, bosses, girlfriends, or lovers more comfortable. At the onset of sexual exploration, being unattached to labels gives you space to dabble with all sorts of pleasures without identifying yourself as anyone other than an explorer! Sexual acts remain pleasure-based, not declarations of solidarity with any group. You decide what you like or don't, try again later and revise your opinion—but avoid getting snared in the limiting tendency to define behavior as lifestyle. Of course, at some point in your progression it might feel quite soothing to wrap a label around you like a cashmere blanket and call it yours. But until that day emerges organically from your experience, labeling denies freedom. Any label to which you one day adhere becomes far more meaningful and certain for having been chosen, not designated.

4. Make Your Desire Rule

The rule to beat all rules is this: Never sex in the absence of desire.

A Babe knows all her desires, actively chooses among them, discriminates among them, knows their signs—mental and physical—and can tell the difference between being horny, hungry, and lonely. She doesn't sex just because she's lonely and she doesn't eat just because she's horny. At least not very often.

Learn the signs that tell you you're hot and hungry for erotic contact, and learn what feeds the need. Learn to tell when you desire to *be* desired, or desire approval, or desire to fit in. Before you get down with anyone, ask: Whom am I trying to please? If the answer isn't "me," ask why not. Always ask, "Who has the power to decide?" If the answer isn't "me," scoop up that power like marbles on the playground and go home. This is how you demonstrate your ability to sustain balance between individuality and connection. If you go out on the prowl wanting to be wanted, stop the game when you win the prize. You don't owe anyone for wanting you. Don't pay them off with your body. If you feel an uncontrollable need to toss your admirer a coin, tell him he's cute and sexy, and get his phone number, just in case—then move on.

> **BABE BOOSTER**
>
> *Learn to say, "OH, that's wonderful!" and "If you touched me just a little higher (slower, to the left) I'll go through the roof!"*

If you're in a relationship, notice when you give in to your partner's desire for you without feeling sharp twinges of desire for him or her. Yes, sometimes it's hot to let his desire drive yours—like lighting a candle from the wick of an already burning one. Sometimes it's even insanely exciting to fuck "cold." It's amazing how a sudden invasion of lust can propel you from zero to sixty in a few seconds. But it's not wise to let a partner's desire rule too often.

Chances are your desire needs to be stoked slowly, so be brazen about showing your lovers how to gingerly bring your arousal to dizzying heights. The Taoists, 3,000 years ago, conceived of women's sexual energy as watery, slow to boil, but able to hold its heat, and men's as fiery, quick to burst into flame, then extinguish. Practitioners of Taoist sexuality today instruct men in bringing the waters of female passion to a gradual boil and women in pleasurably delaying a male partner's incendiary responses. (Taoists, by the way, maintain an almost reverential approach to masturbation.) In honor of this tradition, think about feeling your desire pour from the inside out, not launch from the outside into you.

In my sex therapy practice, I've seen many women substitute being desired for having the experience of desire. Eventually they turn off to sex. Often that's when couples come to therapy together, the guy wondering what happened to his wife's once accommodating libido. In most cases, she never relied on her own libido to drive her sexuality, she relied on his for momentum. She enjoyed sex when she gave in to it, but never found her threshold of active demand. I've had clients who didn't even understand the difference between being desired and desiring. They were often willing to take whatever was offered sexually in the hope that pleasure would follow. They didn't know they could want sex so badly they ached, didn't know they could almost climax from thinking about sex, or could fantasize themselves into spinning around inside like a child's top. That lyric from the old torch song *Black Magic* comes to mind: "I'm "lovin' the spin I'm in." These women wouldn't have understood it. You, Babe, can make that lyric your mantra.

5. Seek Deep Thrills

A Babe's erotic experience is always thrilling, but the thrills are deep, not cheap. Every sexual adventure is potentially an act of creative expansion, but if we don't take good care of ourselves as we tiptoe across the erotic high wire, we run the risk of falling headlong into exploits that leave us feeling used and discarded or fused and out of control.

Some women use sex to fill an amorphous, yawning emptiness that has nothing to do with authentic desire. They use being wanted to salve feeling unlovable, or being degraded to replicate childhood abuse, or being physically hurt to relieve devastating inner pain. Their escapades aren't about sexual adventure any more than stuffing themselves with dry cake mix out of the box is about delectable cuisine. All of these acts are about using intense sensation to cope with indefinable emotions. If you're one of these women, I hope you'll talk to a counselor right away.

A Babe realizes that getting smart about her choices includes paying attention to the difference between real sexual self-expression and stunt-sex to get an adrenaline rush, or opiate-sex to stop hurting. A Babe does not partake of these thrills. Nobody and nothing drives a Babe's sexual choices except her own authentic lustiness mediated by self-knowledge.

Living up to this axiom gets tricky because it means you can't always foretell the nature of a thrill by isolating the particular sexual behavior that produces it. You can't say, for example, that giving nonreciprocal oral sex is always a bad idea, or that reciprocal oral sex is a good idea. (Forgive a tangent here: The trend toward women giving head like good-night kisses is a pet peeve of mine because, in the name of being ever so sexually so liberated, women give while men take, and there's nothing new or liberating about that!) Still, you only know what a behavior signifies *to you* by tuning in to your desire, not his desire, or your desire to be desired, or your desire to please. You know *when* you crave and you know *what* you crave, and you can tell the difference between indecipherable hollowness that begs to be filled up with distractions and true erotic hunger.

One of my clients, Chris, was hooked on chintzy thrills. She spent her weekends chasing after men who would barely give her the time of day. If an unavailable man could be seduced, she felt seen and authenticated.

Chris had been briefly married to a man who was sexually and emotionally inaccessible. He insisted on an open marriage, but spent far more time with his girlfriends than Chris. Since Chris didn't really take to this arrangement but felt powerless to resist, the whole set up was semi-coercive. Chris spent two years trying to lure the man she had married into her bed—two years trying to become real. At just twenty-six, she divorced him, a wise move in itself, except for one small detail—Chris became obsessive in her need to conquer, thus feel acknowledged by, stand-ins for her husband. In her fantasy world, it was her ex who she would use and dump, over and over again. Her life was defined by vengeance and haphazard stabs at acquiring identity through angry sex. Finally, her best friend confronted her with the destructiveness of her actions and Chris wound up in my office. Obviously, there was nothing deep about Chris' thrill seeking.

Deep thrills leave us with a feeling of radiance rather than a backlash of gloom, self-loathing, or despair. Deep thrills contrast with dramatic, cheap thrills in that they offer substantial pleasures and lasting rewards that always outweigh the struggle of acquiring them. The pleasure may be its own reward—like discovering that a fantasy you've harbored for years is even more exquisite in enactment. The delight may be an outgrowth of the achievement in an experience, like feeling proud of yourself for having pushed past your inhibitions to tell a partner what you need in bed at the beginning of the relationship, instead of waiting to feel secure. In our most thrilling moments, pleasure and reward mingle. You reveal what you need and your partner comes through like a champ.

Deep thrills reflect and enhance authenticity. They energize you and bulk up your confidence. Cheap thrills may fill a void, but they leave you stuck in old patterns, erect barriers to intimacy, and obscure your goals. Cheap thrills misappropriate your power, *deep thrills illuminate it.*

Deep thrills are like all the delectable chocolates in the box. Cheap thrills are the empty wrappers, alluring with the scent of sweetness, holding nothing.

6. Accept No Authority but Your Own

A Babe takes her time exploring her erotic universe. She isn't desperate to pile up a lifetime of experiences in her first few months or even years of adventuring. She understands why axioms such as "get your feet wet," and "get your bearings," and "time is on your side" became clichés in the first place. They embody ageless truths. Even her mother knew *those* rules!

It may be tempting to collect all your Babe stripes at once, but the balance and authenticity you're seeking has a developmental schedule of its own. Sometimes less is more and slower really is better. You're in charge of the pacing, and you're in charge of the action. Remember:

- A Babe can as easily say no as yes, yes as no.
- A Babe can stop at any point in a sexual encounter should her desire wane. The word *enough* is rubbed raw from use. She isn't manipulated by males whining of blue balls—she can remain affectionate and relaxed while a guy uses his own hand.
- A Babe can ask for more of what arouses and pleases her and say "no thanks" to anything, anytime. She knows her desires ebb and flow and she surfs them effortlessly. The game that's a yawn today may be a wild ride tomorrow. Hasn't it always been a woman's prerogative to change her mind?
- A Babe realizes that sometimes her lust is purely carnal, unemotional, uncomplicated. Sometimes it reflects a longing for deep, intimate connection. She knows there is fucking and there is making love. She can do both.
- A Babe can operate aggressively out of her power or she can own the erotic act of temporarily giving that power away. Her power belongs

to her, to do with as she pleases.

These points are Babe ideals, but making them realities takes consciousness and practice. Women, raised to please, cooperate, connect, and merge, struggle to delineate sexual boundaries and then police them in ways that men—who grow up with a sense of sexual entitlement—can barely imagine. Policing boundaries is scary. We risk disapproval, desirability, maybe even love. So be it.

Nobody else is going to secure our boundaries for us, and the people we want in our lives are those who admire our ability to conscientiously take care of ourselves.

7. Delineate Boundaries Early in Your Relationships

At the beginning of a potential love affair, every sexual encounter is a field of engagement where boundaries are either breached or preserved. Here is where we set the tone for our role in the budding relationship. Once we set the tone, it's difficult to reset. Best to test your Babe mettle at the outset of a relationship, where you will be meeting challenges to your authenticity, boldness, and balance at every turn. The following story shows how a propitious moment can capture the dynamics of a new relationship and determine its course.

Let's say you're on a second date with someone you're very attracted to. You've had a great night, you're clicking on every level, and after returning to your date's place and making out for a while, you're ready to build on the sexual energy. Some oral delights seem in order and you can't wait to initiate, but you haven't yet had a talk about safe sex. One of your limits is no oral without a barrier. You know some men aren't too thrilled about wearing condoms while you go down on them, so you're prepared for a little resistance. Sure enough, when you pull a silver packet out of your purse and unwrap the contents your date calls a halt.

"You don't need that," he says, "I'm clean."

"I'm more comfortable this way for now," you respond, unwrapping the rubber and preparing to apply it to his pulsating organ.

"I don't feel much with those things on," he protests, and gently but firmly tries to nudge your head down toward his erection, expecting your resistance to crumple like the foil wrapper clutched in your hand.

"Wait, I've got an idea," you offer, ever the optimist. You have your limits, true, but you're also willing to innovate for mutual pleasure. "I'll squeeze some lube inside the condom, and I'll use my hand at the same time as I'm giving you head. I know you'll feel a whole lot more that way." And because you are so well prepared, having perfected this technique over many months, you pull a tiny sample packet of lubricant out of your purse.

"Listen, I really like getting head the regular way," he whispers, his hand now cupping your crotch.

"Have you ever tried it the way I'm suggesting?" you squirm. "Don't spit it out until you've tasted it," you smile weakly, hoping a joke will lighten things up.

His hand leaves its warm niche and settles back into his own lap. "Look, I didn't realize you were so...so...rigid. Maybe this whole thing isn't such a good idea after all."

Uh oh. You offered him a chance to sample your best trick and he turned you down. The whole night flashes before your eyes: his cute smile, his sense of humor, his delicious kisses. Plus, he's smart, successful, and he wants kids someday. He has most of your real-relationship criteria down cold. Could you be making a big deal over nothing? After all, the chances of picking up an STD orally are fairly slim. Granted, you don't know anything about his sexual history, but most of your friends give head without condoms and nothing really bad has ever happened. Maybe you should relax your boundaries with this potential Mr. Right. You don't want him to slip through your eager-to-please fingers.

BABE BOOSTER

Men have hormones, too. Remember: Testosterone is a great equalizer. (It turns all men into morons!)

Your stomach does a summersault. This could be a make it or break it moment for him, and you don't want to blow it.

Actually, this should be a make it or break it moment, but not for him—for you. If you scrap the condom, you'll be telling him that from this time forward he can bully you out of your principles. If that isn't what you want, you'll need to straighten up, take a deep breath, and have a grown-up chat about your concerns. If your date's "my way or the highway" attitude sticks after his brain floats back up to the top of his head where it belongs, there's probably a whole lot more about Mr. Wrong that you don't want to be around long enough to uncover. But let's not put the focus on the questionable stuff he's made of—let's look at what you're made of.

You decided to insist on barrier protection for a good reason, right? You did your homework, and you gave the matter serious thought. If you're willing to negotiate the issue, you owe at least as much time to reconsidering it as you gave to your original decision. A lightening quick turnabout under pressure to appease this man would merely give form to your fears. This is how an obsessive relationship is born—right here—in this first self-sacrificial offering on the altar of insecurity. If you should succumb to your date's need for satisfaction now, and to your own desperate romantic fantasies, your act would be one of renunciation, not gratification. This first of many surrenders would tilt the balance in your relationship, your new lover gaining power from your diminishment. You really have no choice in this predicament—you have to stop the action to preserve your integrity and set the tone for the future.

Whether your boundary is about condoms, or intercourse, or multiple partners, or living out his fantasy, or being punctual, or telling the truth, each time you draw a thick, steady line between what is okay and what is not okay, you are declaring: I belong to me. I am not available to be manipulated by the highest bidder or the one who exerts the most influence or even the one whose rejection frightens me the most. My values are nonnegotiable. I expect them to be respected.

Genuine lack of respect is your signal to exit the situation *fast*. For a Babe, self-sacrifice is never an option. Of course, a lover can only show respect for boundaries that are clearly delineated. If you are vague or wishy-washy, a misstep based on confusion can seem like a deliberate transgression. Part of growing more balanced is learning to be precise about how you communicate your limits. Balance also includes being willing to renegotiate *for cause*. Cause means that the relationship itself has reached a level where you feel safe to relax certain boundaries, or your own perspective has changed as a result of insight or experience. Cause is not "he wants, so I give in."

Taking care of yourself is a way of safekeeping others. By being clear about your own boundaries and limits, you let loved ones know what they can expect from you. Although no one will like all your choices all the time, sincere people will appreciate knowing that your word has meaning. If "no, I won't" is backed by strength, then "yes, I will" carries equally reliable enthusiasm and solidity. A lover needn't fear being unfairly blamed when things don't go perfectly in bed or out, because he knows you take responsibility for all of your choices equally.

When you put faith in your own principles and base your decisions on them, not on whim or pressure, others trust you, too. Your balance and authenticity coalesce into a sturdy platform, a foundation supporting you and those you love.

8. Be Truthful, Accountable, and Responsible

As powerful beings, we have responsibilities to ourselves and to those with whom we are intimate, whether intimacy lasts an hour or a lifetime. Acting from integrity separates Babes from, well, bimbos! The more erotically unconventional you are, the more grounded in well-thought-out values and ethical principles you'll need to be.

Common slight of hand places half-truths and lies of omission at the heart of far too many hurtful episodes between lovers. Think back upon all the times you wondered why someone didn't come right out and tell you:
- He was thinking about seeing other people.
- He didn't want kids.
- He didn't love you.
- He wasn't attracted to you.
- He had ADD.
- He didn't make as much money as you thought he did.
- He was in therapy.
- He was bisexual.
- He had herpes.

And what about all those hurtful tiny withholds?
- He pretended to like your cooking.
- He thought women with short hair looked like dykes, including you.
- He didn't like the way you rubbed his penis.
- He was afraid to play rough with your breasts because he thought your implants might burst.

If you've been hurt even once by a partner's evasion, think for a moment about all the self-disclosures you dodged, too, for fear a lover would be hurt, disapprove, or, worse, take a hike.

Of course, certain intimate secrets should be divulged only on a need-to-know basis. There's no reason to rip your heart out and present the bloody mess on your first date, like a cat with feathers in her teeth plunking a bird at her owner's feet.

> **BABE BOOSTER**
>
> *When you have an important news flash about sex to present to your partner, tell him when you are in a nonsexual situation. Driving in the car together is perfect. There's no sex—and no escape!*

Intimate connections need to be grounded in integrity, and if you are being sexual, you are being intimate. No matter how casual or brief the relationship, it's your obligation to be forthcoming with any information that might contribute to a partner's decision about whether to open him/herself to you or vice versa.

Sex unleashes powerful energies—emotional, sacred, and soulful. Relating to others with love, respecting for their precious humanity, and regarding for their potential vulnerability is a Babe's ethical responsibility.

A Babe does not participate in games where the winner is the one who collects the most used condoms regardless of the human cost!

As a sexual adventuress, you are by definition inviting both emotional and physical risks. Your sense of balance and your core principles need to be especially strong and well conceived to support often unpredictable turns of events. Truthfulness, self-respect, and a willingness to be accountable for your actions are key.

Your personal approach to principled sexual exploration will develop over time, but at the outset you should at least:

- Discuss STDs.
- Use safe-sex techniques.
- Reveal the status of other relationships: yours and your prospective partner's.
- Avoid married or committed lovers whose partners don't condone their sexscapades—it's a surefire way to create havoc in your life, and it's plain bad ju ju!
- Honor all limits of sexual play.

- Talk about whether you're actually dating or merely "playing." This can get muddy, but you can't afford to be squeamish about confronting the matter if there's confusion.
- Clarify needs for afterplay and after-contact, both yours and your partner's.
- Make no promises you can't fulfill.
- Follow through on promises you make.

9. Embrace Taboos

Taboo conjures the glamour of the forbidden, the erotic allure of damned and dark appetites. This book is overflowing with topics, not to mention blatant suggestions, which would be considered taboo among certain circles in the present, as well as among most civilized peoples in the not-too-distant past. Yet, here I am, suggesting that you wrap your arms around taboo like a loved one.

And why not? Sexual excitement, we've learned, is a matter of blending attraction and obstacles. Danger and fear—including the fear of condemnation for having trifled with taboo—is transgressively thrilling. If taboo inspires you—you go, Babe!

Toying with taboo often brings greater depth and excitement to core relationships. Take Andy and Rochelle, for example.

Rochelle was annoyed that her sales executive husband kept hosting clients at strip clubs. She and Andy argued over the matter until, during one tiff, Andy challenged Rochelle to check out the scene before making a fuss.

Rochelle's quick retort: Me? Watch those (perfect, gorgeous, intimidating!) women rub their crotches in your face? I don't think so! But a few weeks later, Andy told her he'd be out with a client at the club and dangled the carrot again. "Why don't you join us," he suggested, just as her eyes began to blaze.

All day Rochelle chewed on the offer and finally made up her mind to give Andy a little surprise.

The real surprise was Rochelle's. Seeing the humor, playfulness, and almost innocent eroticism at the club calmed rather than ruffled her feathers. Randy, thrilled she had come, bought a dance just for her, and being the recipient of the attention gave Rochelle a taste of the harmless excitement the men experienced. As striking as the women were, she realized she wasn't jealous—she saw them as skilled entertainers, like Vegas showgirls up close and personal. A few months later, when a newspaper ad for an exotic dance class appeared, she leaped at the chance to learn a few teasing, pleasing moves of her own.

Embracing taboo helped Rochelle break through an emotional wall and added not just spice, but closeness and fun to her relationship. She often joins her husband at the club now, and it's a perk for his clients to have their voyeuristic tastes further treated when Andy's lovely wife responds so happily to the lap dances he purchases just for her.

That said, consenting grown-ups can embrace any taboo, except one—self-sacrifice.

Forsaking yourself is the only true sin. Its punishment—hell on earth.

10. Be Wary of Confusing Lust with Love

- Sex is not love.
- Sex is activity.
- Sex is energy.
- Sex is sensation.
- Sex is expression.
- Sex is many things, but it is not love.
- Sex can be used, abused, feared, avoided, embraced, refined, disciplined, extolled, debased, and glorified, but sex cannot be transformed into love.
- Only love is love.
- When sex and love coalesce, something brand new is born in the marriage of one with the other.
- Sex can express love, but sex is not love.

You may have noticed that I have scrupulously avoided using the term *fetish* to describe any sexual alternative mentioned so far. Even though fetish is used quite loosely these days in art, fashion, and sex-positive culture, it still carries the pathological connotation of an act or body part *required* for sexual gratification. And because this book is not about pathology, I've steered clear. However, I'm going to break my own rule just to make a point.

I recently took part in a gals gabfest, and the subject of fetish clothing and sexual fetishes came up. We talked about the kind of quasi-fetishistic needs we each had, or at least were willing to admit. One woman revealed that she couldn't climax unless her boyfriend pulled her hair. Another needed to hear her lover moaning in order to orgasm. But in the end we all agreed that women have one truly perverse craving—if we can be said to be universally fetishistic about anything, it's that many splendored thing, that thing that makes the world go round, that crazy thing called love.

If we couple our love fetish with the granules of shame that we just can't get one hundred percent out of our psyches—a bit like the last remaining grains of beach sand in our sneakers—we discover a confusion of lust with love that gets us in a heap of trouble.

There are countless ways in which we create havoc by mistaking lust for love. But they all begin and end with failed attempts to make the self *we really are* congruent with the self *we think we ought to be*, and in so doing, we sacrifice our authenticity.

Authenticity demands savage honesty in the plodding, unsparing investigation of ourselves. None of our lies about love or lust can survive if we are relentless in asking "who am I, *really?*" as we take each step forward in life. A Babe always asks that question.

Intimate relationships demand the same code. The exploration of our inner mysteries, undertaken in stereo with a beloved, forces encounters to their truest, riskiest levels. The joy of long-term love is in penetrating each other's hearts, scouring the depths of each other's erotic souls. Magic isn't found in some unchanging formula for mere pleasing, satisfying sex, but in the endless uncovering and discovering of the person within, going always farther, higher, always hazarding more. If digging into ourselves alone is frightening, then the archeology of love is only more so. Yet, as we develop the willingness to mine all that is real inside us—especially in the tantalizing danger zone of our erotic world—we are preparing for partnership.

In the deep quarry where hearts converge, our lessons in being a Babe ground us. They confer the power and wisdom that enable us to weather the storms of love and celebrate its immeasurable joys.

All your lessons in becoming a Babe are really lessons in becoming resilient and whole. Buoyed by the erotic, the creative, the authentic, you sprout wings.

Step out now, Babe, and release your irrepressible spirit. You know you're oh so ready to fly.

Afterplay

The following resources are organized according to the chapter of this book in which they were originally mentioned or to which they most directly relate. This is not meant to be an exhaustive list and it reflects only some of my personal favorites. Many of the Web sites listed also carry links to other recommended sites or to outstanding and comprehensive bibliographies. For example: http://www.sexuality.org/sexbib.pdf.

Web site descriptions reflect the nature of the site as this book went to press, but the cyber universe is ever changing, so approach judiciously.

Foreplay

Muscio, Inga. *Cunt: A Declaration of Independence*. Seattle: Seal Press, 1998. If I had a daughter, this book would be the jumping-off point for many heart-to-heart talks about what it means to be a woman in today's world. Muscio's jewel belongs on the same shelf with classics such as *Our Bodies, Ourselves*.

Chapter 1: The Fine Art of Becoming a Babe

Winks, Cathy and Semans, Anne. *The New Good Vibrations Guide to Sex: Tips and Techniques from America's Favorite Sex Toy Store*. 3rd Ed. San Francisco: Cleis Press, 2002.

Truly an everything-you-ever-wanted-to-know book about female sexuality with an empowering, dare-anything edge. One of the few sex bibles around, and my personal favorite.

Chapter 2: The Roots of Romantic Obsession and Chapter 3: Overcoming Romantic Obsessions and Setting Yourself Free

Engel, Beverly. *The Emotionally Abusive Relationship: How to Stop Being Abused and How to Stop Abusing.* New York: John Wiley & Sons, 2001.

Engel, Beverly. *Loving Him Without Losing You: How to Stop Disappearing and Start Being Yourself.* New York: John Wiley & Sons, 2002.

Beverly Engel is a terrific writer and therapist who knows what sets healthy relationships apart from the "other" kind. Both of these books are gems.

Gilbert, Roberta. *Extraordinary Relationships: A New Way of Thinking About Human Interactions.* New York: John Wiley & Sons, 1992.
The nuts and bolts of Murray Bowen's "differentiation theory" in the first 150 pages. Recommended for those who like the basics minus long-winded storytelling.

Lerner, Harriet. *The Dance of Anger: A Woman's Guide to Changing the Patterns of Intimate Relationships.* New York: Harper and Row, 1985.

Lerner, Harriet. *The Dance of Connection: How to Talk to Someone When You're Mad, Hurt, Scared, Frustrated, Insulted, Betrayed, or Desperate.* New York: Quill, 2002.

Lerner, Harriet. *The Dance of Intimacy: A Woman's Guide to Courageous Acts of Change in Key Relationships.* New York: Perennial Library, 1989.

No mincing words, Harriet Lerner is a national treasure. Her books are smart, real, and insightful. To my knowledge, she was the first to use the term "self-focus" in popular writing and, from my point of view, deserves the credit for coming up with a user-friendly way of referring to Bowen's concept of differentiation.

Schnarch, David. *Passionate Marriage: Keeping Love & Intimacy Alive in Committed Relationships.* New York: Owl Books, Henry Holt & Co., 1998.
From his vantage point as a sex therapist, Schnarch addresses key issues in self and relationship development. I don't agree with everything Schnarch has to say, but there is much good stuff to be mined. Seekers of the quick fix will be disappointed; depth-seekers won't be.

Chapter 4: Release the Shame, Unleash the Slut

Damsky, Lee, Editor. *Sex and Single Girls: Straight and Queer Women on Sexuality.* Seattle: Seal Press, 2000.
For six months I kept this book on my nightstand and read essays at random. Each is a superb glimpse of a woman grappling with her heat, her heart, and the thicket inside her head.

Chapter 5: Your Erotic Seventh Sense

Bright, Susie. *Full Exposure: Opening Up to Your Sexual Creativity and Erotic Expression.* San Francisco: Harper, 2000.
Bright's passionate essays will challenge, enliven, and inspire women and men alike.

Ogden, Gina. *Women Who Love Sex: Enhancing Your Sexual Pleasure and Enriching Your Life.* New York: Pocket Books, 1994.
Based on groundbreaking research, women who celebrate their erotic selves share their stories.

Chapter 6: Kindling Erotic Fantasy

Britton, Patti. *The Adventures of Her in France.* Beverly Hills: Leopard Rising, 2001.
Britton is a sexologist (ivillage.com's in-house sex coach) and, as this book attests, a talented writer of sizzling erotica. The fantasy in Chapter Six entitled "Love's Surrender" was adapted from this book. Available at http://www.yoursexcoach.com.

Daniell, Rosemary. *Confessions of a Female Chauvinist.* Athens, Georgia: Hill Street Press, 2001.

Daniell, Rosemary. *Sleeping with Soldiers: In Search of the Macho Man.* New York: Holt, Rinehart, Winston, 1984.
Daniell is one true Babe who weaves stories of her iconoclastic life with literary skill.

Morin, Jack. *The Erotic Mind: Unlocking the Inner Sources of Sexual Passion and Fulfillment.* New York: Harper Collins, 1995.
Research-based, fascinating, and powerful exploration of Eros' beguiling, irresistible allure.

Rainer, Tristine. *The New Diary: How to Use a Journal for Self-Guidance and Expanded Creativity*. Los Angeles: Jeremy P. Tarcher, Inc., 1979.
Thoughtful, comprehensive, with lots of imaginative techniques and an excellent chapter on eroticism.

WEB SITES

American Association of Sex Educators, Counselors, and Therapists
http://www.aasect.org
Should you have any serious concerns about the nature of your fantasies or any other aspect of your sexual experience, it's best to speak with a counselor. I advise seeing a certified sex therapist who is also a licensed psychotherapist. Referrals to practitioners throughout the country are available at the AASECT Web site. In addition to AASECT, skilled therapists can be found through the America Board of Sexology at http://www.sexologist.org.

Blue Door
http://www.bluedoor.com
At this site, you can rent adult films discretely through the mail. Selection runs the gamut and includes extreme hard-core, sensual, "women friendly," and sex education titles.

The Erotica Readers and Writers Forum
http://www.erotica-readers.com
Have you ever thought about writing an erotic story? This site is a writer's wish list come to life—everything but the paycheck! Also a great spot if you just enjoy reading gifted erotic writers or are seeking new erotic visions.

Femme Productions
http://www.royalle.com
Producer/Director Candida Royalle's movies are sensuously explicit but skip the gynecological close-ups and "money shots" common to traditional adult films. Her style reflects what women want while also appealing to the more enlightened man. Available for rent or purchase at video stores, via the Web site, or at 1-800-456-LOVE.

Libido: The Journal of Sex and Sensibility
www.libidomag.com
The original literary journal has gone online, offering resources across a wide swath of the sexual universe. I love the feminist perspective on sexual history and current events, plus fiction, new books, and the showcasing of independent video documentaries and erotica. A must-see!

Chapter 7: Cultivating Self-Pleasure and Self-Love

Abrams, Douglas; Abrams, Rachel Carlton; Chia, Mantak; and Chia, Maneewan. The *Multi-Orgasmic Couple: Sexual Secrets Every Couple Should Know*. San Francisco: Harper, 2002.
This contains the secrets of ancient Taoist sexuality. Valuable depiction of how women's sexual responses and needs differ from men's and how to achieve powerful pleasure—regardless of the number of orgasms.

Ladas, Alice Kahn; Perry, John; and Whipple, Beverly. *The G-Spot*. New York: Dell, 1983. This is the classic, popular explication of Grafenberg's work and subsequent discoveries about the eponymous spot.

Morin, Jack. *Anal Pleasure & Health: A Guide for Men and Women*. 3rd Ed. San Francisco: Down There Press, 1998.
Yes, this is everything you ever wanted to know and then some. Safety, psyche, sensuality, hygiene, how-to—the works.

WEB SITES

Babeland (a.k.a. Toys in Babeland)
http://www.babeland.com
Great Web site for sex toys, crystal wands, erotic accessories, books, movies, and explicit sexuality information. You can find stores in Seattle and New York. This friendly, knowledgeable staff will present a paradise for Babes!

Good Vibrations
http://www.goodvibes.com
The first, and still one of the best, pleasure stores for women in the nation, stockpiled with every sexual accoutrement imaginable.

The G-Zone: Tools and Education for a Better Sex Life
http://www.doctorg.com
Sexologist and researcher Dr. Gary Schubach's Web site, full of sources for information on the G-spot and female ejaculation. If you want to understand the science of female pleasure, this is a good place to begin.

House O' Chicks
http://www.houseochicks.com
The home of the wondrous vulva puppet, a beautiful, handmade velvet vulva representation that is both a one-of-a kind work of art and a sex education aid. Vulva University offers a dozen online classes in the erotic arts—from advanced alternative sex play to Tantra and Sex Toys 101. Also available, free postcards featuring the stunning visual art of Yuri Shiller.

Libida: Sex Toys, Tips, and Erotica for Women
http://www.libida.com
One-stop shopping for toys, videos, books, articles, stories, and more—it's all here!

Natural Contours
http://www.natural-contours.com
Candida Royalle's site for her own line of sleek, sexy vibrators made to fit a woman's curves and for use solo or during lovemaking for that extra zing.

Real Women Project
http://www.realwomenproject.com
The Real Women Project uses sculpture, poetry, video, music, and storytelling to inspire women's self-acceptance and broaden our definition of beauty.

More sites for women's erotica, resources, and links
http://www.cleansheets.com
http://www.scarletletters.com
http://www.femmerotic.com

Chapter 8: Pure Exposure, Extreme Eroticism

Anapol, Deborah. *Polyamory: The New Love Without Limits: Secrets of Sustainable Intimate Relationships.* San Rafael: Intinet Resource Center, 1998.
This is the first popular book on the subject. Not to be missed if you're seriously interested in exploring poly (because you should read everything!), but if you're vaguely curious, see below.

Devon, Molly and Miller, Philip. *Screw the Roses, Send Me the Thorns: The Romance and Sexual Sorcery of Sadomasochism.* San Francisco: Mystic Rose Press, 1995.
Written from a female submissive-male dominant perspective. Highly informative, yet uproariously funny in squashing stereotypes and putting clueless top-dog wannabes in their places.

Easton, Dossie and Liszt, Catherine A. *The Ethical Slut: A Guide to Infinite Sexual Possibilities.* San Francisco: Greenery Press, 1998.
The personal experiences of the authors contribute to a fascinating read. For my money, the better overall intro to the subject.

Easton, Dossie and Hardy, Janet. *The New Bottoming Book.* San Francisco: Greenery Press, 2001.

Easton, Dossie and Hardy, Janet. *The New Topping Book.* San Francisco: Greenery Press, 2003.
Exceptionally frank, friendly, and knowledgeable guides to the art and skill of playing on either side of the bdsm divide. Easton is a licensed therapist in San Francisco and Hardy also writes as Catherine Liszt, co-author of *The Ethical Slut.*

Munson, Marcia (Editor) and Stelboum, Judith P. (Editor). *The Lesbian Polyamory Reader: Open Relationships, NonMonogamy, and Casual Sex.* New York: Harrington Park Press, 1999.
In my opinion, this is the most powerful book on polyamory, and the material applies regardless of one's sexual orientation. The complexities and pitfalls along with the delights are realistically exposed in a series of essays offering a broad perspective.

Wiseman. Jay. *SM 101: A Realistic Introduction.* San Francisco: Greenery Press, 1998.
Essential for your S&M starter kit!

WEB SITES

The Institute for 21st Century Relationships

http://www.lovethatworks.org

Small but growing, grassroots organization offering support for and education about all forms of ethical, consensual relationship styles.

Loving More

http://www.lovemore.com

Publisher of *Loving More* magazine, dedicated exclusively to topics involving multipartner relating. Distributes poly-relevant books, hosts conferences and workshops, and acts as a national clearinghouse and public forum for the polyamory movement.

On Our Backs: "The Best of Lesbian Sex"

http://www.onourbacksmag.com

Newsstand magazine goes online with articles and stories. Totally hot stuff whether you're hetero, bi, lesbian, or simply have a pulse.

MATCHMAKING WEB SITES

Consider this a sampling of sites, each with its own cache and peculiarities. Since you can browse them for free, look long and well before you leap.

General dating sites

http://kiss.com

http://match.com

Personals at http://yahoo.com

Personals at http://nerve.com

Alternative, Sex-Oriented, or Kinky Matchmaking

http://alt.com

http://bondage.com

http://adultfriendfinder.com

Chapter 9: Babes in Action

Ensler, Eve. *The Vagina Monologues*. New York: Villard, 1998.
The show is a phenomenon and if you don't see it performed, you're missing out on a cultural revolution. In any case, you can still read the book!

Klein, Marty. *Beyond Orgasm: Dare to Be Honest About the Sex You Really Want*. Berkeley: Celestial Arts, 2002.
A solid book about sexual honesty and intimacy that you can share with loved ones.

WEB SITES
How to Be a Babe
http://www.howtobeababe.com
Where else would you expect to find more for Babes? Check it out!

The Society for Human Sexuality
http://www.sexuality.org/
Possibly the best sexuality resource on the Web. Its range of topics and articles seems boundless.